Plant-Based Meal Preparation Cookbook

Ready to go Meals and Snacks for Organic and Healthy Plant Based Eating and Vegan Diet with Over 100 Recipes to Prep Your High Protein Low Carbs Keto Meals

By

Adele Tyler

All trademarks and brands within this book are for clarifying purposes only and are the owned by the owners themselves, not affiliated with this document.

Table Of Contents

Introduction

A plant-based diet is a diet that includes foods mostly or only from plants. People use various ways of describing the term plant-based diet. Some vegetarians describe it as a vegan diet that includes foods avoiding all animal products.

Consumable food in a plant-based diet

A plant-based diet means plant foods, such as fruits, vegetables (like spinach, kale, zucchini, cauliflower, Brussels sprout,), whole grains, nuts (like peanuts, almonds, and walnuts), seeds (like chia seeds, flax seeds), coconut oil, olive oil, and legumes. A plant-based diet focuses on whole foods that are organic, rather than refined.

Foods to avoid

You have to avoid foods like beef, pork, eggs, chicken, turkey, duck, crabs, fish dairy products, and ice-creams, gelatin, and honey.

Health Benefits of plants based diets

Plants based diet has more benefits than weight loss; it reduces your blood pressure. It balances cholesterol levels and keeps your heart healthy. It prevents you from type 2 diabetes. It also helps in reducing weight and help you to live long. Plants based diet prevents certain types of cancer. It has many benefits for athletes and old people.

Vegan keto diet

A vegan keto diet is the combination of a vegan diet and a keto diet. Keto diet involves cutting your carbs and depending on fats for your energy. Keto diet involves proteins from animal sources, but a vegan diet restricts it. So when you are on a vegan keto diet, you take protein from various other sources like tempeh, vegan eggs, tofu, seitan, and vegan protein powder.

The fat requirements are fulfilled with nuts, coconut oil, olive oil, vegan cheese, and coconut yogurt.

Chapter 1: Introduction to Organic and Healthy Plant-Based Eating

1.1 What Is a Plant-Based Diet?

Plant-based or plant-forward eating patterns focus mainly on foods prepared from plants. This includes not only vegetables and fruits but also nuts, seeds, oils, whole grains, legumes, and beans. It doesn't mean you're vegetarian or vegan and don't eat meat or milk. Instead, you select more of your foods regularly from plant sources.

 Much research on nutrition has looked at plant-based eating patterns such as the Mediterranean diet and a vegetarian diet. The Mediterranean diet has a basis of plant-based foods; it also includes few times a week fish, poultry, eggs, cheese, and yogurt, with less frequent meats and sweets.

The Mediterranean diet tends to lower the risk of heart disease, metabolic syndrome, diabetes, cancers (specifically colon, breast, and prostate cancer), depression in large population and a decreased risk of frailty in older adults, along with better mental and physical health.

It has also been shown that vegetarian diet supports health, including a reduction in risk of having coronary heart disease, high blood pressure, diabetes, and an increase in a long life.

Plant-based diets provide all the protein, fats, carbohydrates, vitamins, and minerals required for optimal health, and are often higher in fiber and phytonutrients. Some vegans might need to add a supplement (specifically vitamin B12) to ensure they get all the nutrients they need.

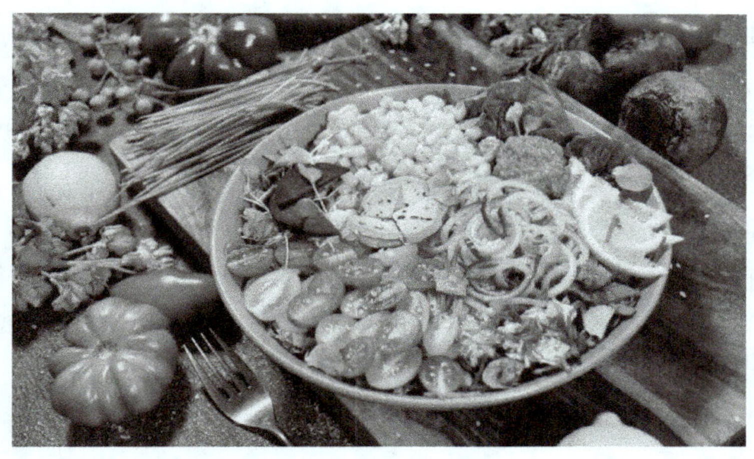

Ways to start plant-based diets

Here are a few suggestions that will help you start a plant-based diet.

Eat a lot of vegetables

Dinner and lunch, fill half of your plate with vegetables. Make sure you pick your vegetables with plenty of colors. Enjoy the vegetables with hummus, salsa, or guacamole as a snack.

Pick good fats

Especially safe options are the fats in olive oil, olives, nuts and butter, seeds, and avocados.

Cook at least one or two vegetarian meals a week

Make beans, whole grains, and vegetables around those meals.

For breakfast, include whole grains

Start with the barley, quinoa, buckwheat, or oatmeal. Then add some fresh fruit along with some nuts or seeds.

For dessert, eat fruit

After a meal, a ripe, juicy peach, a refreshing slice of watermelon, or a crisp apple will fulfill the urge for a sweet snack.

Go greens

Every day, try a variety of green leafy vegetables like kale, collars, Swiss chard, spinach, and other greens. Heat, barbecue, boil or stir-fry to retain the nutrients and flavor.

Have a meal built around a salad

Fill a bowl with romaine, spinach, bib, or red leafy greens. Add a variety of other vegetables, including fresh herbs, beans, peas, or tofu.

Change your way of thinking about meat

Take smaller quantities, instead of taking a centerpiece take it as a garnish.

1.2 Benefits of Plant-based Diet for Athletes

Athletes are always in search of a competitive edge – and this might mean swearing off meat. Elite Olympians-NFL linebacker's athletes are following vegan or vegetarian diets for better results, quicker recovery, and overall safety.

- The athletes are at risk for heart disease: 44 percent of professional cyclists and runners have coronary plaques according to a study. A plant-based diet protects the hearts of athletes by removing the plaque, raising blood pressure and cholesterol, and weight loss.
- Consumption of meat and high levels of cholesterol intensify inflammation, which can lead to pain and weaken athletic performance and recovery. Studies show a diet based on plants can have an anti-inflammatory effect.

- Plant-based diets maximize arterial strength and flexibility, resulting in improved blood flow. Even a single high-fat meal, like Mc muffins has had several hours of impaired arterial function.
- A plant-based diet contains saturated fat and free from cholesterol, helps improve viscosity or thickness in the blood. That allows the muscles to get more oxygen, enhancing athletic performance.
- Plant-based diets can lower your body fat because it is typically low in fat and high in fiber. Reduced body fat is linked with increased aerobic capacity — or the ability to fuel exercise using oxygen. Research shows that athletes on a food intake based on plants increase their VO2 max — the maximum supply of oxygen they can use during high-intensity exercise — resulting in better endurance.
- People eating a plant-based diet are getting more antioxidants compared to meat-eaters, which help neutralize free radicals. Fatty acids lead to fatigue in the muscles, decreased athletic performance, and impaired recovery (Esposito, 2019).

1.3 Benefits of Vegan Lifestyle for Old People

Potential benefits to seniors taking a vegetarian diet

There are indeed a number of ways in which an older adult could benefit from a vegetarian diet.

Slow aging

A plant-heavy diet can increase telomerase activity, which are the enzymes found at the end of a human DNA that reconstructs telomeres.

U.S.-led research Department of Defense has found that a plant-based diet can significantly increase our telomeres' activity, which in turn can help slow down the effects of the aging process. It has been found that processed meat has just the opposite effect, shortening telomeres over time.

Reduces stress

A vegetarian diet can lower your cortisol levels, which is a stress-related hormone.

Improves skin

The antioxidants found in plants help to moisturize the skin, heal the skin tissue, and remove premature aging molecules.

Energy boost

Energy is connected to our digestion process. Since breaking down plant foods is easy for a senior's digestive system than meat, a vegetarian diet can provide more energy all day long. And boosting energy is critical to getting some daily exercise for older adults, and maintaining a happy and healthy lifestyle.

Peaceful sleep

Bananas, sweet potatoes, kale, and nuts are all high in vitamin B6, magnesium, and tryptophan. These important vitamins and minerals help increase melatonin and create a healthy cycle of sleep, which is particularly important for the health of senior citizens.

Boost brain function

A plant-based diet can help minimize the risk of cognitive disorders such as Alzheimer's and vegetables like broccoli and cauliflower have properties that can improve brain activity and help you think more clearly.

Tips for aged vegetarians

One possible risk of switching to a vegetarian diet is protein loss. Protein is very important to a senior diet because they tend to lose muscle mass as they age, and it is necessary to get enough protein to help their bodies build muscle.

There are plenty of protein sources which vegetarians can eat, for example:

- Yogurt (Greek)
- Eggs
- Cottage cheese
- Peanut butter
- Black beans
- Sunflower seeds
- Milk
- Lentils
- Oats

As long as you eat protein from other sources, the adverse effects of taking meat out of your diet can be minimized.

1.4 Importance of Plant-Based Eating in Daily Life

A plant-based diet is often proclaimed as the healthiest eating approach, and its benefits extend far beyond weight loss.

Registered dietitians, as well as food scientists, have been praising the benefits of eating plants and cutting back on meat for years. And people are seemingly switching on. A study released in The Permanente Journal in the summer of 2016 states that plant-based diets have gone mainstream — partially because the advantages. The healthcare professionals support eating this way because they have seen excellent outcomes.

Going plant-based is not so much a diet as a general eating method. There is no need to count calories or stress every day to meet certain macronutrient goals. Essentially, it's just about eating more plant-based foods (and fewer animals-based foods while you're at it).

A diet based on plants can keep your heart healthy.

Meat contains saturated fat, which can lead to heart problems if consumed excessively. So by cutting meat and loading up on plant-based foods, you're doing your ticker a favor. A study published in August 2019 in the American Heart Association found that eating a plant-based diet may decrease the risk of having the cardiovascular disease by 16 percent and dying of this health condition by about 31 percent.

But it's not just about restricting meat — you have to make sure that the plant-based foods that you consume are safe instead. According to a study in 2017 in the American College of Cardiology, this means eating whole grains, legumes, vegetables, fruits and healthy oils (such as olive oil) rather than unhealthy plant foods, such as refined grains and sugary beverages, which may increase your risk of heart problems.

A diet based on plants can reduce your blood pressure.

According to the doctors committee, high blood pressure, or hypertension, can increase the risk for health problems like heart disease, stroke, and type 2 diabetes. Luckily the food you eat will make a difference.

Several studies have shown that sticking to a plant-based diet will reduce blood pressure and thus reduce your risk for those conditions. A meta-analysis published in Internal Medicine in April 2014 analyzed data from 39 studies and found that, on average, people who followed a vegetarian diet had lower blood pressure than those who followed diets based on animals.

Type 2 diabetes prevention

It is well known that diet and type 2 diabetes are related. Weight is a big risk factor as more fatty tissue makes the cells more resistant to insulin, according to the Mayo Clinic. But which type of diet is best suited to prevent type 2 diabetes? Studies say a plant-based one has advantages. A study published in 2016 in PLoS Medicine found that eating a plant-based diet filled with plant foods lowers the risk of developing type 2 diabetes by 35 percent. The American Diabetes Association states that it is likely that plants are lower in saturated fats than animal foods that raise cholesterol levels and the risk of developing type 2 diabetes. Another study in Diabetes Care found the occurrence of type 2 diabetes was 7.7 percent among non-vegetarians and only 2.8 percent for vegans.

Help you reduce Weight

Your risk of obesity reduces when you swap a meat-based diet for a plant-based one. In short: Plant eaters tend to weigh less, even if the No. 1 goal is not always that. "The idea is to feed the body and cells in order to improve health outcomes, but weight loss could be a by-product of replacing and reducing certain foods," says Feller.

Helps in Longer Life

All the other potential benefits listed here are rolling into one big one: to live longer. A study by the American Heart Association Journal found that a plant-based diet reduces the risk of all mortality causes by 25 percent. And beyond that, if you stick to safe plant-based foods, the protective levels increase. A study published in The Journal of Nutrition in April 2018 found that eating healthy plant foods versus unhealthy foods extends the protective layer by another 5 percent. In order to identify healthy plant foods, researchers assigned a score between 1 and 17 to various non-animal products. Less healthy foods — such as soda, coke, and white bread — were given a low score, though free of meat; meanwhile, healthier plant foods — such as whole grains, veggies, and fruit — were given a higher score;

Diets with lots of fruits and vegetables, particularly leafy greens, carrots, pumpkin, and sweet potatoes, may help prevent age-related macular degeneration from occurring.

Improvement in the cholesterol level

High cholesterol can lead to fatty blood deposits that can limit blood flow and potentially lead to heart attack, stroke, or heart disease. But a balanced diet can aid in reducing cholesterol levels. In particular, moving away from a diet filled with animal products to one based primarily on plants can reduce LDL ("bad") cholesterol by between 10 and 15%, while those following a strict vegan diet can reduce their LDL cholesterol by as much as 25%, according to a study published in The American Journal of Cardiology.

Arthritis

Eliminating dairy consumption has long been linked to alleviating the symptoms of arthritis, but a new study indicates that a combination of a gluten-free and vegan diet is very promising to improve the health of those with arthritis.

Reduce the cancer risk

As we have shown, there are many health benefits of eating a plant-based diet — but does it help prevent cancer? Research indicates Yes may be the solution. The American Institute for Cancer says eating a diet rich in vegetables, fruit, grains, beans, nuts, seeds, and some animal foods are the safest way to source cancer-protective nutrients, including fiber, vitamins, minerals, and phytochemicals. And the same applies to those who survive cancer. A review published in 2011 in Cancer Management notes that there are protective benefits, although they are moderate (lowering the risk of certain cancers by about 10 percent) and are likely due to the nutrients in plant foods, and eating this way promotes a healthy weight (Lawler, 2020).

1.5 Best Plant-Based or Vegan Foods to Consume

Food you can eat

In a vegan or plant-based diet, you can eat foods made from plants, including:

- Legumes such as beans, lentils, and peas
- Nuts and seeds
- Bread, rice, and pasta
- Vegetables and fruits
- Vegetable oils
- Soymilk, almond milk, and coconut milk

Foods to avoid

Vegans or plant-based eaters are required to avoid any foods made from animals, including:

- Beef, pork, lamb, and other red meat
- Chicken, turkey, duck, and other poultry
- Shellfish such as crabs, mussels, and fish
- Eggs
- Cheese, butter

- Milk, ice cream, cream, and other dairy products
- Mayonnaise (because it includes egg yolks)
- Honey

Chapter 2: Meal Prepping Using Plant-Based Ingredients

2.1 Importance of Meal Prepping

A healthy lifestyle, living life full of energy attracts all of us. Lets face it, and life can be busy! While setting healthy eating goals may be easy, it can be tricky to follow through with those goals and stay consistent.

The idea of cooking all of your own meals at home can sometimes feel impossible when you're busy going through your daily life. Avoiding all of the restaurant temptations and let's face it- a time when it comes to deciding on a meal is the number one "make or break" factor.

If you're sick of spending too much money on restaurants and not meeting your fitness goals, meal planning is your new best friend.

'Meal prep' is the process of arranging, preparing, and packing your meals and snacks in advance, usually for the coming week, with the goal of clean eating and managing portions. It is a secret that helps a lot of people meet their fitness and health goals.

Remember that there is no wrong or correct way to prepare meals, as it is all about what works for you personally. The ultimate goal is to save time in the kitchen over the week and to have access to healthy meals. Some people will find that they like to prepare their weekly breakfast, lunch, and dinner while others will only prepare one meal for each day.

Is meal preparation really so scary in advance? Maybe the fear emerges when you imagine your whole Sunday in the kitchen being destroyed by cooking, or maybe you're afraid if you have to eat from the same large batch of turkey all week, your meals will be boring and tasteless. Doesn't it? Well, could you just be afraid of failure, knowing planning ahead isn't your strong suit?

The fact is, if you prepare meals properly, none of those worries can come to fulfillment. Of course, as the saying goes, planning to fail is a failure to plan. Whether you're serious about weight loss, muscle packing, or just adding more vegetables to your life, then the Holy Grail is meal planning.

Recognize and address the weak spots —

The meals or snacks that need the greatest attention, like if you eat out every night, then start preparing with dinner. If, after your morning workout, you are unable to figure out what to take as a proper breakfast, start with your post-workout meal.

Set aside some time for initial preparing and cooking, and you'll be surprised at the many advantages that meal preparation has to bring.

You will save more money

When you plan in advance, then you will know exactly what do you need for the coming week. When you buy things in bulk quantities, it will cost you less, thus saving your money and also stops you from going to the market again and again to buy things. So meal prepping will save your money and time also. You only need to invest some time in advance to plan your meals and cook them. A lot of times we spend at the fridge trying to figure out what to cook.

Meal prepping saves wastage of food

Have you ever had to throw away items that went bad before you had an opportunity to eat them? It does not feel good. You use all of your ingredients for the week when you start preparation, and it is very unlikely that if you plan correctly, you will have any leftovers!

The grocery will become easy for you

When you know what meals you're going to eat for the week, shopping at the grocery stores should feel like a breeze! Forget about walking aimlessly around the store. Take your list and split it into categories such as fruits, vegetables, protein, frozen foods, milk products, grains, and fats. Also, it will help you avoid the areas you don't need to go to, like the candy area.

It will increase your will power

As you switch your eating habits and start eating healthy food regularly, you'll slowly stop hunger for sugar and other fattening ingredients. Keeping a routine in place is important to eat healthily, and you'll find it easier to stop eating foods you know you shouldn't eat!

It lowers your stress

Stress can affect the immune system, leading to digestive disorders, and interrupt sleep patterns. It can be frustrating to come home from work and start preparing your dinner. With meal preparation! You can say goodbye to the tension of "what's for dinner" and knowing that your meal just needs a little heating.

It will give you a variety of food

If you can think ahead of time about your meals, choosing from several different food categories (protein, fat, grains, vegetables, etc.)It will become easy to get the variety you need to give to your body. Only feel free to mix it every week! You're not going to be limited to the simple foods you make out of habit as the meal planning allows you to become more experimental by looking up new recipes.

It' helps in weight loss

Planning your meals beforehand is important for weight loss because you know exactly what you put into your body and how much. A weekly meal plan routine allows you to monitor how many calories you add on a daily basis, which is the ideal weight loss formula.

Teach you the art of portion management

The beauty of meal preparation is that you will learn balance. Bringing your meals in containers will prevent you from taking more quantity of food. If you are going to lose weight and consume the right amount of nutrients, controlling portions is very important. You can give yourself treats from time to time, but it is important to control how much you consume.

Keep in mind, there is no bad or correct way to achieve a routine meal prep. People have their own style of doing it, and you will begin to realize through trial and error what works best for you and what doesn't! (SCHILDHOUSE, 2020).

2.2 Planning for Multiple ready to go Recipes

List of Common Ingredients Required for Recipes

Nuts

- Almonds*
- Brazil nuts
- Hazelnuts/filberts
- Macadamia nuts
- Pecans
- Peanuts*
- Pine nuts*
- Walnuts

Seeds

- Hemp seeds
- Chia
- Pumpkin
- Sunflower

Butters

- Hazelnut butter
- Almond butter
- Macadamia
- Coconut butter
- Peanut butter
- Pecan butter
- Sunflower seed butter
- Tahini Walnut butter

Oils

- Avocado oil
- Cacao butter
- Flaxseed oil
- Hazelnut oil

- Macadamia nut oil
- Olive oil
- Almond oil
- Coconut oil

Fruits and vegetables

- Artichoke hearts
- Arugula
- Avocados
- Blueberries*
- Coconuts
- Collards
- Asparagus
- Endive
- Celeriac
- Bell peppers
- Spinach
- Brussels sprouts*
- Cabbage
- Carrots
- Cauliflower
- Celery
- Broccoli
- Rutabaga
- Chard
- Beets
- Fennel
- Fiddleheads
- Jicama
- Kale
- Eggplant
- Kohlrabi
- Lettuce
- Cucumbers

- Mustard greens
- Okra
- Onion
- Garlic
- Radishes
- Rhubarb
- Mushrooms
- Shallots
- Swiss chard
- Turnips
- Zucchini
- Cranberries
- Lemons
- Olives
- Watermelon
- Raspberries
- Strawberries
- Tomatoes

Pantry Staples

- Baking powder
- Artichoke hearts
- Coconut flour
- Coconut milk
- Baking soda
- Coca or cacao powder
- Almond flour
- Dark chocolate (85% and up)
- Jackfruit (green, canned in brine)
- Psyllium Husk
- Nutritional yeast
- Vanilla extract

Herbs and spices

- Edamame

- Kelp noodles
- Kelp flakes
- Lupine beans*(p)
- Nori sheets
- Roasted seaweed
- Shirataki noodles

Sauces & Condiments

- Chili sauce
- Hot sauce
- Hummus*
- Mustard
- Soy sauce/tamari
- Salsa
- Tomato sauce
- Vinegar

Fridge Staples

- Apple cider vinegar
- Dairy-free yogurt*
- Dairy-free cheese*
- Pickles
- Sauerkraut
- Seitan*(p)
- Sprouts (all kinds)
- Tempeh (p)
- Tofu (p)

2.3 Reusing the Ingredients in Different Dishes

You should get creative! You can store vegetable trimmings and bones in a stock bag, and store them in the freezer. You'll be able to use these remaining vegetables and bones into homemade stock once the bag is full. Stale bread or even bread can end up turning you into breadcrumbs. And if you're making stuffed zucchini boats, you can add the inner parts of the zucchini you're not going to use to bulk up a frittata instead.

If you only have one or two vegetables to get used to, try making a pureed soup with them:

Chop the ingredients approximately (include onion and a few garlic cloves if you have them), sauce them with a spoonful of canola or olive oil and some salt, and pour in enough stock to cover the ingredients. Bring to boil and cook for at least 10 to 20 minutes, then simmer.

Puree

An immersion blender is a great pureeing tool and season your soup however you'd like. Or keep it easy with a tiny butter, so it feels rich and special.

Fried vegetables

When roasted, all the vegetables shine, the high temperatures bring out the natural sugar content of a vegetable, which creates beautiful flavor.

Caramelized color and taste.

Just toss with a little oil, salt and pepper at the most basic. Try one of our favorite flavor here for a little extra credit. If you roast more than one vegetable and if the cooking time really varies, separate it into two sheet pans or start the longer-cooking one first and then add the others later in the roasting process.

Curry (Thai)

Like stir-fries, any vegetable combination will blend into the bold aromas of delicious curry. A couple of spoons of curry paste and some coconut milk will turn your spoiling cabbage, peppers, carrots, squash, and so on into something wonderful.

2.4 Equipment Required for Meal Prepping

Food processor

Without any hiccups, it can chop, shred, julienne, and slice batches of vegetables. It will mix ingredients into smooth nut butter, soups, sauces, and dips easily. It can shred cheese in seconds and make bread crumbs. Actually, it will do everything you need — and fast. You might spend half an hour chopping mushrooms or carrots for the week at your kitchen counter, or you might have this food processor do it in seconds.

A sheet to bake

A baking sheet is an excellent gadget for baking veggies, cooking proteins, making entire one-pan meals, baking desserts, and much more. You could toss a mélange of vegetables on this like Brussels sprouts, potatoes, and carrots roast them all at once and then make portions of them for a week's meal.

Instant Pot

In a slow cooker, you set your meal, and you can press a button when you go out, and when you came back home, you have your food ready to eat. The Instant Pot works faster as it is a pressure cooker and is just as useful. The gadget has a kind of cult following and can be used to make large batches of oatmeal, rice, yogurt, and chili, as well as whole roast chickens and a small family's worth of veggies.

If you'd like to minimize your time in the kitchen for preparing your meal, the Instant Pot is definitely the way to go.

Containers

Once you've cooked your meals, you'll need to make its portions and put them into containers that are easy to transport and durable. Compared to conventional Tupperware containers, the collection of steel containers is an unusual option, but it is extremely helpful for meal preparation. It comes as a stack of three or two, so you can separate foods that might get soggy; the bottom of each container serves as the lid for the one on top, and for easy portability, there's a lid with a carrying handle.

A Crock-Pot

Crock-Pot meals mean you'll be in the kitchen for as little time as possible. If you have to make large quantities of soups and stews or the creamiest cheese and mac, the Crock-Pot slow cooker is your best tool. You can make countless dishes with this kitchen wonder, and once you get the hang of it, you won't believe you've ever lived without it (Bratskeir, 2020).

2.5 Storing and Reheating Prepared Food

Tips for Freezing Food

Using freezer in your kitchen will not only bring some peace of mind to your meal preparation but will also help foster healthier eating habits by making nutritious, homemade meals readily available during times when you're hungry and want a quick and easy dinner option.

It is important to allow pre-cooked foods to cool down before putting your dish into the freezer, as putting a hot dish in your freezer would lower the total freezer temperature, which may contribute to the defrosting and spoilage of foods around it. If you're in a hurry, instead of using the refrigerator to quickly cool down dishes — which will lead to the same problem but with your refrigerated foods — give them an ice bath in the sink. Put water in your sink and some ice for this method, and lower your hot dishes into it for a couple of minutes, making sure the water reaches just halfway up the sides of your platter.

Use airtight containers when freezing food. Airtight lidded plastic containers should be frozen to reduce the amount of outside oxygen flowing into the bowl. It's also advisable to double-wrap your plastic containers in a freezer-proof plastic wrap layer if you're planning more than a week of storing the dish.

When freezing casseroles, it is always best to opt for a shallow casserole dish, which will result in a faster process of reheating, as well as better heat distribution throughout the entire dish.

Make sure to completely wrap the entire container to limit the oxygen flow when storing bigger dishes and casseroles. Start by covering the top of the dish entirely with freezer-proof foil, and then wrap the whole dish in plastic wrap. The addition of the second layer of plastic wrap will result in fresher flavors with no risk of freezer burning, depending on the length of time you plan on storing it.

Meals names should be written on all containers, the date it was prepared, and detailed reheating instructions before being stored away. This will ensure that the food is eaten within a safe period of time, and that other family members will be able to properly reheat the dish if you are not around to help.

When freezing cooked meats, fruits, grains, and pasta, it is prudent to only tender slightly undercook before freezing. When reheated, each of these ingredients will cook slightly more so they can easily become overcooked if well-done is stored.

Make sure that the temperature of the freezer is low enough while your dishes are cooling, the prepared food should be placed at 0 degrees Fahrenheit in your freezer.

Reheating tips

In order to make sure that your prepared food is safe for your future use, food should always be defrosted in the refrigerator rather than at room temperature.

To thaw a prepped casserole safely, switch the dish to the refrigerator 24 hours prior to cooking. Cook the casserole at the same temperature as originally requested by the recipe, adding an extra 15-20 minutes to the time, and occasionally checking the plate temperature.

The microwave can be an easy thawing and reheating method for those in a rush (if the portion size is right). If using a microwave — or high-capacity toaster oven — it is wise to use a thermometer to measure from time to time the temperature in the center of the dish to ensure a safe 160 degrees Fahrenheit is reached.

You can directly put your food from the freezer to the oven when you reheat a pre-cooked casserole. Cook the dish at the same temperature as you would if it were fresh to cook, but give the dish and extra 20 minutes, checking the dish's progress intermittently to make sure it heats properly, but not overcooking.

Keep the foil layer in place when heating a casserole dish in the oven, fold back the corner or cut a couple of slits in the top to allow steam to be released from the platter. During the heating, rotate the dish periodically to allow for reheating (Houston, 2018).

Chapter 3: Sweet and Salty Breakfast Recipes

3.1 Vegetarian Cheese Quiche Stuffed Peppers

These cheesy peppers stuffed with quiche are an easy brunch or an easier breakfast. A lightly seasoned filling of the eggs is made fluffy with a mixture of full-fat ricotta, mozzarella, and shredded Parmesan bite. It takes only a few leaves of fresh spinach to give those beautifully colored peppers a little green boost! The steps are so simple that in minutes you can throw this down together and have it in the oven. Just mix the filling and pour it over the prepared peppers, cover with foil, and bake. The next day they are great to reheat too.

Ingredients

- Two flax eggs (add 1tbsp.flax seeds with 3 tbsp. water)
- Half cup ricotta cheese
- Two medium bell peppers, cut from the center and remove the seeds
- Half cup shredded mozzarella
- Half cup grated Parmesan cheese
- one-fourth tsp. dried parsley
- One teaspoon garlic powder
- One fourth cup baby spinach leaves
- Two tablespoons Parmesan cheese, to garnish

Instructions

Heat oven to 375°F. Shape the peppers by cutting them into equal parts and take out the seeds.

In a food processor, mix the three pieces of cheese, eggs, garlic powder, and parsley. , or you can do this in two batches, half and half, and then join the fillings.

Add the egg mixture in the peppers, filling them just under the rim. Put some spinach leaves on top and mix it with a fork, pushing them down the egg. Cover all the peppers with foil and bake for 36-46 minutes or till the egg is set.

Put with Parmesan cheese and broil for 3-5 minutes or until the tops begin to brown.

This makes a total of four single-servings of Vegetarian cheese quiche Stuffed Peppers. Each serving comes out to be 245.5 Calories, 5.97g Net Carbs 5.97, 17.84g Protein and fat 16.28

3.2 Asparagus and Tomato Frittata with Dill and Havarti

Asparagus and tomato frittata with dill and Havarti is a great spring breakfast when asparagus begins to go on sale, and if you don't have Havarti to make this tasty frittata.

This Asparagus and Tomato Frittata with Havarti and Dill is a great thing to make for breakfast, lunch, or dinner.

Ingredients

- Six oz. fresh asparagus trim ends and cuts it into small pieces
- Two teaspoon olive oil
- 2/3 cup chopped cherry tomatoes
- One tsp. dried dill weed or (two tsp. minced fresh dill)
- Four oz. Havarti cheese, cut into cubes.
- Six eggs beat them well.(or use flax eggs)
- Spike seasoning and Vege-Sal to taste the eggs add some salt and fresh-ground black pepper or all-purpose seasoning of your choice if you don't have Spike.
- Chopped green onions for garnish (optional)

Method

Cut off the asparagus spears' woody ends, then cut asparagus into pieces about 1 1/2 inches in length.

Heat olive oil on a medium flame in a frying pan, add asparagus and cook for 3-4 minutes.

While cooking asparagus, dice the cherry tomatoes to half (or fourths if large) and dice the cheese into small pieces.

After cooking asparagus for 3-4 minutes, add the cherry tomatoes and dill weed and cook for another 1-2 minutes.

Break eggs in a bowl, then beat well.

When tomatoes have cooked for 2 minutes, pour them over the eggs, season with Spike Seasoning and Vege-Sal or black pepper salt and fresh ground, then sprinkle over the end. Some pieces of asparagus and tomatoes will poke up at this point, but the frittata will puff more as it cooks.

Start the broiler with preheating.

Cover pan and cook about 8-10 minutes at low heat, or until the eggs are set, and the cheese is completely melted on top.

Put frittata under the broiler for a couple of minutes, carefully testing to see when it would start to get brown.

Slice the frittata into four wedges, garnish with sliced green onions and serve hot when the top is browned to your liking (DENNY, 2018).

3.3 Sweet Potato Black Bean Burritos

Those sweet potato vegans and black bean burritos are a great breakfast choice. The beans offer meaty texture while the sweet potatoes are silky and buttery.

Time to prepare: 10 minutes

Cooking time: 30 minutes

Total time: 40 minutes

 Serving: 6

Ingredients

- Two tablespoons olive oil

- One cubed sweet potato

- One tablespoon of chili powder

- Half tsp salt

- Half tsp paprika

- Half tsp of garlic powder

- One fourth tsp cumin

- One-fourth tsp pepper

- Rinsed and drained one can of black beans

- Six tortillas, medium shaped taco

- 1/4 Cayenne Powder

- One cup Salsa, Divided

Method

Preheat oven to 400 degrees. Mix the sweet potato cubes, paprika, olive oil, pepper, chili powder, cumin, garlic powder, salt, and cayenne together in a medium bowl. Spread the sweet potato mixture onto a baking sheet in one even layer and bake for 25 minutes.

Add the black beans onto the hot baking sheet when the sweet potatoes are cooked, and mix them together.

Assemble the burrito by placing into the center of a tortilla half cup sweet potato and black bean filling. Even pour one tablespoon of salsa over the mixture of sweet potatoes, and roll the tortilla into a burrito.

Upon assembly of all the burritos, heat up a large skillet over medium heat. When the pan is hot, put each burrito down into the seam of the skillet. Brown for about 2 minutes, then turn the sides of the burritos and brown for a further 2 minutes.

Serve with Cilantro and Salsa (Hungry, 2018).

3.4 Blueberry Quinoa Breakfast Bars

These easy, quinoa breakfast bars are packed with protein and whole grains, naturally sweetened, gluten-free, and contain zero oil or butter.

Ingredients

- One and a half cup cooked quinoa (about half cup dry)
- One flax egg
- one tsp ground cinnamon
- One-fourth tsp kosher salt
- half tsp baking soda
- 1 1/4 cups fresh blueberries
- one tsp baking powder
- 1 cup milk (non-dairy milk)
- One and a half cups rolled oats
- Half cup unsweetened applesauce
- One fourth cup maple syrup
- Three tbsp. almond butter — or nut any butter
- One tsp vanilla extract

Method

Put your baking tray in the middle of the oven and preheat to 350 degrees F. Brush gently with spray-on an 8-inch square non-stick pan. Place a parchment paper so that the opposite sides of the paper overhang like handle the edges of the pan. Spray non-stick spray to the parchment paper.

Mix together the oats, cinnamon, quinoa, baking powder, salt, and baking soda in a medium bowl (It is suggested to use a rubber spatula and to move the ingredients gently until they are uniformly blended for easier combination because the quinoa will be a little moister). The milk, applesauce, almond butter, maple syrup egg, and vanilla are mixed in a separate large cup.

Place the dry ingredients into the wet mixture and blend to stir. The batter is going to be very moist. Fold in the blueberries, then pour into the baking tray.

Bake for 38 minutes or until golden brown, thickened and dense, and a toothpick inserted in the middle of the **quinoa**, it comes out clean. Using the parchment paper as handles, immediately lift the bars out of the pan and transfer them gently to a wire rack. Let it cool, cut into bars, and serve.

3.5 Overnight Vanilla Breakfast Oats

Missing your bowls of oat filled up overnight? If so, this keto-friendly, low-carb, paleo version of the "overnight oats" will be best for you! Those grain-free breakfast bowls, made perfect with Hemp Hearts, are a total win. Simply soak overnight and enjoy in the morning, adding an extra milk splash before eating.

Prep time: 5 mins

Total time: 5 mins

Serves: 2

Ingredients

- One tbsp. chia seeds

- half cup hemp hearts Manitoba harvest

- Two tsp of confectioners erythritol or three drops of stevia liquid

- Half tsp vanilla extract

- Two-third cup coconut milk

- Himalayan salt a pinch

- Optional Toppings

- Six raspberries whole

- Twelve almonds whole

Method

Mix in all ingredients into a 12fl Oz (350 ml), or larger box with a cap. Cover and set overnight in the refrigerator for at least 8 hours.

Add extra milk the next day until target consistency is reached.

Divide between two small cups, add toppings, and enjoy if desired.

Variation: Overnight "Oats" in Keto Fudge Add 2 tablespoons of cacao powder and one tablespoon of sunflower oil, in addition to the ingredients in the Vanilla version above. Follow the directions set out above. Shredded unsweetened coconut, cacao nibs, and strawberries are optional toppings.

Store in the fridge in a container for up to 2 days for possible leftovers.

3.6 Blueberry Oatmeal

Blueberry baked oatmeal recipe is a delicious, easy, and healthy breakfast packed with protein with no added sugar! Topped with fresh blueberries and sweetened with keto maple syrup, these blueberry oatmeal bars are vegan and gluten-free!

Preparation time: 5 minutes

Cooking time: 20 minutes

Total Time: 26 minutes

Ingredients

- Half cup almond butter
- Two cups oats rolled, gluten-free
- keto maple syrup
- Half cup blueberries
- One fourth cup mix-ins of choice

For the glaze

- Coconut milk half cup
- Half cup powdered sugar-free sugar

Instructions

Oven preheats to 180C/350F. Line an 8 x 8-inch parchment-paper pan and set aside.

Combine all your ingredients in a large mixing bowl, except for the blueberries, and mix well. Use a spatula of rubber to fold the blueberries in half. If the batter is too thick to thin out, add some milk. Add some extra oats if the batter is too thin.

Move the batter to the recessed plate. Place remaining blueberries on the top and bake for 20-25 minutes, or until they are golden and the center comes out just clean.

Remove from the oven and allow the oatmeal baked with blueberry to cool in the pan for 15 minutes, before being carefully transferred to a wire rack to cool completely.

When cold, drizzle the sugar-free icing over them.

Use nuts, white chocolate chips vegan or seeds

3.7 Peanut Butter Chia Pudding

Chia pudding makes not only a delicious vegan keto breakfast but also a delicious vegan snack or vegan keto dessert.

This delicious vegan keto breakfast pudding is made the night before and is a simple way to make breakfasts for you. Before eating this amazing chia pudding, make sure you allow at least 3 hours to blend flavors in the fridge!

What makes this pudding keto like a sweetener is the combination of chia seeds, almond milk, and sugar-free monk fruit.

Preparation time: Ten minutes

Time to cook: Three hours

Ingredients

- Peanut butter one cup no added oil, no added sugar

- One and one-fourth cup unsweetened almond milk - I used Almond Breeze

- Chia seeds grounded one fourth cup

- 1/4 teaspoon salt

- Monk fruit pure extract three drops

- Vanilla essence one teaspoon

- liquid sweetener of choice or powdered erythritol or one fourth cup maple syrup sugar-free

Topping tips

- The peanut butter one teaspoon

- Crushed peanuts half teaspoon

- Sugar-free dark chocolate one teaspoon

- Chocolate chips sugar-free one teaspoon

Method

In a blender blend, all the ingredients and the order doesn't matter.

Mix for 30 seconds, stop and scrap the blender's side and bottom with a spatula. Blend for 35 seconds-1 minute, or until smooth and creamy.

At this stage, it is recommended that you check the sweetness and adjust for a sweeter pudding with extra drops of monk fruit extract (or stevia drops). You can also boost the sweetness with extra maple-flavored syrup, but the pudding will change the texture, the more syrup you apply, and the more liquid the pudding will become. That is why it is preferred to use drops to adjust the sweetness.

Transfer into eight small glass jars, 1 serving approximately 1/3 cup (80ml)

Refrigerate for the best creamy texture and flavors, for at least 3 hours.

Serve with optional toppings. Recommended sugar-free dark chocolate chunks, chocolate-free melted sugar drizzle, peanut butter drizzle, and crushed peanuts.

Place it in the refrigerator in a container for five days.

3.8 Tofu Scramble

High in protein and amazing eggy vegan tofu scramble! This tasty and enjoyable vegan breakfast is real close to scrambled eggs in texture without truly being scrambled eggs, which would be extremely awesome! Ideal for vegans who miss eggs and for those who want a tasty, healthy breakfast.

Ingredients

- 8oz (~220g) Extra Firm Tofu
- Vegan Butter one teaspoon
- Paprika half teaspoon
- Turmeric half teaspoon
- Nutritional yeast two tablespoons
- Dijon mustard one teaspoon
- 1/2 tsp Garlic Powder
- Black salt one fourth teaspoon
- one fourth tsp Onion Powder
- one third cup Soy Milk

For Serving:

- Black Pepper
- Fried Tomatoes
- Chopped Chives

- Sliced Avocado

Method

Chop the tofu with a fork and end up leaving some nice large pieces.

Add the nutritional yeast, paprika, onion powder, Dijon mustard, turmeric, garlic powder, black, and salt to a medium bowl. Then add in it the soy milk and whisk it in, so you have a good sauce.

Add the plant-based butter to a frying pan and heat until hot. Place the tofu, fry it until it gets lightly brown. When moving it around the pan, be careful not to break it.

Put in the sauce and roll it in. Fry it until you get the needed consistency; the sauce will be absorbed by the tofu so you can have it as dry or as wet as you like.

Finish with some black pepper and chopped chives and serve with some fried tomatoes and sliced avocado.

3.9 Breakfast Bagels

Preparation time: 10 minutes

Cooking time: 40 minutes

Total time: 50 minutes

Yield: Six vegan keto bagel thins

Ingredients

- flax seed ground half cup
- tahini half cup
- One teaspoon baking powder
- psyllium husk one fourth cup
- water one cup
- Salt a pinch

- Sesame seeds for garnish optional

Method

Preheat your oven to 375Ferenhite.

Add psyllium husk, baking powder, ground flax seeds, salt in a mixing bowl and whisk until thoroughly combined.

Add water in the tahini and mix it well until combined.

Mix together all the wet and dry ingredients and then knead to form the dough. It's important that everything is kneaded thoroughly and that the dough is uniform!

Form patties by hand that are about four in diameter, and one-fourth thick. Lay it on your baking tray and cut a small circle from the middle of each round. Use the bigger end of a large pastry tip that would normally use for piping frosting. A doughnut pan can be used for this step, which makes everything so much easier! Add those sesame seeds now

Bake it for around 40 minutes until it gets golden brown.

Cut it in half, and toast like you would make a normal bagel and enjoy.

Top as desired!

3.10 Breakfast Cinnamon Muffins

Low carb cinnamon muffins gave a keto, and vegan makeover! These super fluffy and bakery-style muffins use almond flour and have no eggs and no butter, but super moist — grain-Free, Gluten-Free, sugar-Free, and dairy-free.

Preparation time: 5 minutes

Cooking time: 15 minutes

Total Time: 20 minutes

Servings: 21 muffins

Calories: 112kcal

Ingredients

- almond butter, sunflower seed butter, peanut butter or any nut or seed butter half cup
- Almond flour half cup
- Coconut oil half cup
- Vanilla protein powder two scoops
- Baking powder one teaspoon
- Cinnamon one tablespoon
- Pumpkin puree half cup can sub for unsweetened applesauce or mashed cooked sweet potato

For the glaze

- Milk one fourth cup
- Coconut butter one fourth cup
- lemon juice two teaspoon
- granulated sweetener one tablespoon

Instructions

Preheating your oven to 350 F and place a muffin tin with muffin liners and place aside. This can also be done by using a mini muffin tin. Combine your dry ingredients in a large bowl and mix well. Put the wet ingredients and mix until combined. The cinnamon roll muffin batter should be evenly distributed amongst the muffin liners. Bake for 10-14 minutes, checking around the ten-minute mark by placing a skewer in the middle and seeing if it comes out clean. If it does, it means muffins are ready. Allow resting in the pan for five minutes to cool before transferring them to a wire rack to cool completely.

Make your glaze by mixing all ingredients well until combined. Drizzle the glaze over the muffin tops and allow them to firm up.

These cinnamon muffins can be kept in the fridge. At room temperature best to use within two days

3.11 Almond Butter Pancakes

Course: Breakfast

Cuisine: American

Yield: 1 batch of pancakes

Calories: 260

Fats: 20.8g

Carbs: 5.1g net

Protein: 9.6g

Fiber: 8.8g

These low carb vegan gluten-free pancakes are the perfect breakfast for your family. They're dairy-free, sugar-free, egg-free, and soy; also, they are high in protein, fiber, and omega-3 fatty acids. The perfect keto pancake!

Ingredients

- Two tablespoons almond butter unsweetened
- Coconut flour one tablespoon
- Salt a pinch
- One-fourth cup of almond milk
- Flax one tablespoon grounded
- Baking powder half teaspoon
- Liquid stevia optional

Method

Take a pan and heat it on low, medium flame. Add some oil in the pan of your choice

Mix almond milk and almond butter in a bowl.

 Combine all the dry ingredients in another bowl and mix well until they are blended well.

Mix together all the dry and wet ingredients, and mix well until they are thoroughly mixed. Let this sit for five minutes, so the coconut flour and flax can absorb the liquid.

Place the batter into the skillet and spread gently into pancakes.

Approximately make four pancakes out of this. If the batter is hard to spread, wet the back of a spoon and use it as a spatula.

Cook for about 4-5 minutes, until the pancake flips (check it by gently putting your spatula under the pancake). Like with conventional pancakes, you want to see those tiny bubbles on the surface.

Cook them for another three minutes until done.

3.12 Cinnamon and Pecan Porridge

Preparation time: 5 minutes

Cooking time: 15 minutes

Nutrition (per serving)

Net 5.2 grams carbs

Protein13.8 g

Fat51.7 g.

582 Kcal Calories

Ingredients

- One-fourth cup of coconut milk

- One tbsp. (15 ml) extra virgin coconut oil or MCT oil

- Two tbsp. (20 g/0.7 oz.) of hemp seeds

- Three fourth cup (180 ml/ 6 fl. oz.) of unsweetened almond milk

- One fourth cup almond butter, roasted preferably (63 g/2, 2 oz.)

- Two tbsps. of whole (16 g/0.5 oz.) chia seeds

- One-fourth cup (28 g/1 oz.) chopped pecans or walnuts

- 1/4 cup of toasted, coconut flakes (15 g/0.5 oz.)

- Cinnamon: half tsp

- Optional: 5-10 drops of stevia fluid

Directions

Mix the almond butter, coconut milk, almond milk, coconut oil in a small saucepan and bring to a simmer over medium heat.

Turn the heat off once hot.

Add chia seeds, chopped pecans, hemp seeds, and toasted coconut (reserve the topping with some coconut).

Add the cinnamon, and add stevia as an option. Mix for 5-10 minutes, and let it rest.

Spoon the porridge into bowls to serve. Hot or cold to drink.

Top with the remaining coconut just before serving, and enjoy!

3.13 Granola

Servings: Fifteen persons

Total Carbs: 3%

Proteins 12%

Equipment

- Baking sheets silicon
- Measuring cups and spoons

Ingredients

- Flaxseeds 60grams
- Coconut oil 50 grams melted
- sunflower seeds hundred grams
- pumpkin seeds hundred grams
- walnuts chopped 70 grams
- cinnamon grounded 100 grams
- ginger grounded one teaspoon
- coconut flakes or chips 250 grams
- four tablespoons of sweetener granulated

Directions

Place all the coconuts, nuts, and seeds in a big, high-sided roasting or baking platter.

Melt the coconut oil and add the ginger and cinnamon. Add sweetener if needed. This is entirely optional and may be a useful addition to starters.

Pour over the granola mixture without grain and thoroughly toss with a large spoon or spatula. Make sure the oil and spices are all fine coated.

Bake for 20 minutes, at 180C/350F.

The mixture is very easy to burn, so turn the mixture with a large spoon, after every three minutes.

Let the granola cool and put in airtight containers.

3.14 Vegan Quiche Cups

Preparation time: 10 minutes

Cooking time: 30 minutes

Total time: 40 minutes

Ingredients

- One tbsp. lemon juice

- 3.5 cups leafy greens of choice

- One block extra firm tofu (14 oz.)

- Three tbsp. water

- ketchup one tablespoon

- Cornstarch one tablespoon

- Nutritional yeast half cup

- Two teaspoon garlic seasoning

- Two tbsp. Dijon mustard

These super-simple vegan quiche cups are totally delicious! They are so easy to make the perfect vegan breakfast or brunch recipe. They're also gluten-free, low-carb, keto, low-fat, oil-free, dairy-free, and low-calorie!

Method

Preheat your oven to 350 Fahrenheit, line muffin tin with non-stick muffin liners or spray with non-stick cooking spray, and place aside.

In a blender, combine all ingredients except leafy greens, and mix until smooth. Add some more water if necessary to facilitate blending.

Pour the blender contents into a large mixing bowl, add the leafy greens, and stir.

Put it into a muffin tray and bake for thirty minutes or until the edges start browning.

Calories 57Calories from Fat 18

3.15 Bulletproof Coffee

Serves: Two cups

Preparation time: 3 Minutes

Total time: Three minutes

You'll love this bulletproof, coffee it tastes better than any other thing! This keto bullet coffee recipe is for a rich and creamy drink using coconut oil, almond butter, and cocoa butter. Making this homemade, bulletproof coffee takes just six minutes.

Ingredients

- One ounce of organic cocoa butter raw
- Two tablespoons of coconut oil, organic and extra virgin
- One-fourth cup of oat milk
- Two tablespoons of almond butter made from 100% roasted almonds
- Two cups of coffee

Method

Heat the cocoa butter, coconut oil, and almond butter in a large jug in the microwave until it melts, for nearly twenty seconds. Add in the oat milk and heat until it gets hot, about thirty seconds long. Add in the coffee and mix until creamy, with a handheld milk frothier or a small blender. Pour into two mugs, and immediately serve.

Because cocoa butter is sold differently and varies in size, if you don't have a scale, imagine it will be two tablespoons when melted.

3.16 Curried Tofu Scramble Recipe

This high-protein curried tofu scramble recipe is a simple and quick breakfast that your whole family will enjoy. It' is filled with onions, peppers, mushrooms, and tons of curry flavor.

Cooking time: 20 minutes

Tofu Pressing Time: thirty minutes

Total Time: 30 minutes

Servings: four persons

Ingredients

Tofu -

- Mushrooms six oz. chopped
- Red pepper one chopped
- Spinach, kale and arugula two cups chopped roughly
- Sodium vegetable broth or olive oil three tablespoons
- Onion one medium chopped
- Firm organic tofu pressed and drained one block

Curry Seasoning Mix -

- Garlic powder half teaspoon
- Half teaspoon curry powder
- Half teaspoon cumin
- turmeric one fourth teaspoon
- Coriander one fourth teaspoon
- Garam masala one fourth teaspoon
- paprika one fourth teaspoon
- Water one tablespoon
- Himalayan pink salt one fourth teaspoon

Directions

Sauté the onions in a vegetable broth in a large saucepan for 5 minutes. Add in red peppers and the mushrooms and cook it for ten minutes.

Place the veggies to one side of your pan and add the tofu block (drained and pressed) on the other side of the pan and use a wooden spatula to break it up into small pieces. Sauté for about three minutes.

Add all the seasonings in a separate bowl and add enough water to mix it together. Pour over the tofu pieces and toss until each piece is coated. Mix up the vegetables and the tofu.

Add the vegetables, cover the saucepan, and cook for five more minutes or until the vegetables become soft. Serve hot and top with hot sauce and green onions!

3.17 Green smoothie bowl with almond butter

Preparation time: 10 Minutes

Full time: 10 Minutes

In this hearty meal, the nutritious combination of protein and healthy fats will set you up for a successful day and avoid the cravings of mid-morning donuts or bagels.

Serves: 2

Ingredients

- One Cup simple dairy-free yogurt Greek

- Eight ounces of spinach or kale

- 1/4 cup of water or unsweetened milk-free drink

- One third Cup Protein Powder

- 1/4 cup almond butter, peanut butter or nut-free sunflower seed butter

- Fresh or frozen strawberries: 1/2 cup

- Two Sprinkled almonds or sunflower seeds

- Two Tablespoons of flaxseeds grounded

Directions

Put the vegetables, protein powder, mix protein powder, Greek yogurt, water, or milk beverage in your blender with nut or seed butter.

Blend until creamy and smooth.

Divide the smoothie into two bowls.

Sprinkle 1/4 cup of strawberries over each smoothie bowl, one tablespoon of almonds or sunflower seeds, and one tablespoon of flaxseed.

3.18 Muesli Low Carb Keto Cereal

Quick and tasty breakfast recipe

Preparation time: 5 minutes

Cooking time: 8 minute

Ingredients

- pumpkin seeds one cup

- pecans half cup

- vanilla extract half teaspoon

- Sunflower seeds one cup

- Coconut flakes unsweetened one cup

- Almonds chopped half cup

- Hemp hearts half cup

- Two teaspoons cinnamon

- One fourth teaspoon vanilla stevia drops or sweet leaf stevia

Method

- Add all the above ingredients in a large mixing bowl and mix them well.

- Place the mixture on a baking tray and bake for eight minutes at 350f.

- Take out from the oven and let it cool.

You can also add some almond milk in it if you like. Eat fresh or pack it in an airtight container.

3.19 Omega 3 Keto Porridge

Preparation time: 5

Cooking time: 3

Total time: 8 minutes

Yield: 1 1x

Category: Breakfast

Ingredients

- Two ounces hemp hearts
- One tablespoon whole or ground raw pumpkin seeds
- Half teaspoon chia seeds
- One-fourth cup of almond milk
- One teaspoon shredded coconut
- 1/8 teaspoon fine sea salt
- Half teaspoon ground Ceylon cinnamon, divided
- 1/4 cup coconut cream, room temperature
- One teaspoon powdered stevia

- Liquid stevia four drops

- Six walnut halves, chopped

Method

Combine the cinnamon in a bowl with the hemp hearts, pumpkin seeds, chia seeds, and salt.

Whisk the coconut cream in a separate bowl with almond milk. Pour the mixture of seeds and stir to combine. Place it in the fridge and chill overnight.

Heat the porridge in the pan on low to medium heat for four minutes when ready to serve, until it is warmed up. Alternatively, heat up for one minute in the microwave.

Mix in the remaining cinnamon, liquid stevia, and stevia powdered to tailor the sweetness to your taste. If needed, a thinner consistency adds more milk.

Cover with walnuts and shredded coconut and serve.

Chapter 4: Vegan Keto Lunch Recipes

4.1 Kale Tofu Stir Fry

This simple fry tofu stir recipe is so easy to make, and a delicious dish ready in 10 minutes or less!

Total time to cook: 10 minute

Serving: three persons

Ingredients

- One block extra firm tofu, cubed
- One Tbsp. sesame seeds
- Six cups chopped kale
- One minced garlic clove
- Two tablespoons soy sauce or liquid amigos

Method:

1. Tofu drain: Let the tofu drain for about 15-20 minutes by wrapping the block of tofu in a paper towel.

2. Spray non-stick cooking spray on the pan. Add minced garlic and bring heat it on a medium flame.

3. forming an even layer add Tofu and cook for two minutes.

4. Add in liquid amino and kale and cook for 9 to 10 minutes, stirring periodically.

5. Top with sesame seeds and serve.

4.2 Tomato Cucumber Salad

A quick and easy salad, you can prepare and pack it in the box for your lunch at your work.

Preparation time: 10 minutes

Total time: 10 minutes

Serving: 4 persons

Calories 176 kcal

Ingredients

- One English cucumber
- One lemon, juiced
- fresh cilantro or parsley two tablespoon
- One green bell pepper
- Half cups cherry tomatoes chopped
- Two ripe avocados chopped
- Red wine vinegar one tablespoon
- Avocado 1/8-1/4 cup or your favorite oil
- pepper and salt to taste

Instructions

Chop the vegetables and remove all the seeds or stems or any skin.

Mix the oil, pepper, lemon juice, vinegar, salt, and fresh herbs of your choice and pour over salad. Mix it well.

4.3 Cauliflower Wings

Make delicious air fryer cauliflower wings with this simple and quick recipe.

Preparation time: 5 minutes

Cooking time: 24 minutes

Total time: 29 minutes

Servings: 4 persons

Calories: 48kcal

Ingredients

- Almond flour one tablespoon

- Salt to taste

- Three to four tablespoons of hot sauce.

- Avocado oil one tablespoon

- One medium head of cauliflower cut into pieces washed and fully dry.

Method

- Preheat your air fryer to 400F / 200C

- Mix together almond flour, hot sauce, salt, and avocado oil in a large bowl.

- Add the cauliflower and mix it well.

- Add the cauliflower but half into the air fryer and fry for fifteen minutes until crisp at the edges.

- Shake the basket of the air fryer halfway thru to turn the cauliflower. Take out and place aside.

- Add in the next batch, but cook it for three minutes less than the first batch.

- Serve and enjoy.

- They can be eaten cold with some extra hot sauce for dipping at your workplace.

4.4 Spinach, Olives and Tempeh Salad

Preparation time: 10 to 15 minutes

Total cooking time: 10 minutes

Ingredients

- One cup frozen spinach

- about six large olives (or more, usually more)

- Almonds one tablespoon chopped

- One cup broccoli florets
- Three ounces tempeh chopped
- Olive oil, pepper, salt, and garlic powder to garnish!

Method

Basically, the process for all of this is sauté in a pan until vegetables are cooked. Season it with salt, chili, garlic, and olive oil.

Lower heat is ideal for keeping oil intact. Add the salsa sauce on it. Spinach is super low in carbs and is generally high in proteins.

4.5 Cucumber Salsa

Servings: 15 people

Calories: 10kcal

Ingredients

- Tomatoes chopped two medium
- Jalapeno peppers chopped and seeded four medium
- Two medium cucumbers peeled, chopped and seeded
- 1/2 medium red onion chopped
- One clove garlic minced
- Lime juice two tablespoons
- Fresh parsley finely chopped two teaspoons
- Cilantro fresh finely chopped two teaspoons
- Half teaspoon salt

Instructions

Take a large bowl, and mix all the above-mentioned ingredients, serve with tortilla (low carb).

4.6 Sesame Ginger Walnut and Hemp Seeds Lettuce Wraps

Preparation time: 10 minutes

Total time: 10 minutes

Servings: Four

Calories: 382kcal

Ingredients

Sauce

- Maple syrup one tablespoon
- Ginger minced one tablespoon
- Toasted sesame oil one teaspoon
- Two tablespoons tamari low sodium, gluten-free
- Brown rice vinegar two tablespoons

Filling

- Hemp seeds half cup
- 2 Dates chopped two
- lettuce leaves
- walnuts one cup chopped
- 1/2 cup chopped cucumber
- Sesame seeds optional
- One-fourth cup chopped carrots

Method

Mix the ingredients to make the sauce.

Add chopped hemp seeds, walnuts, dates, cucumber, and carrots. Refrigerate them for an hour for the ingredients to mix.

Take lettuce leaves and a Pile mixture on them. Top with sesame seeds, if wanted.

4.7 Empanadas

Preparation time: 30 minutes

Cooking time: 10 minutes

Total time: 40 minutes

Serves: 8 empanadas

Ingredients

- Coconut flour half cup
- Cold margarine cubed one fourth cup
- Water four tablespoons
- Two tablespoons tomato sauce
- Half cup almond flour
- Two tablespoons psyllium husk
- One pinch of salt
- 1/2 cup tvp, tofu or seitan
- One teaspoon soy sauce
- 1/2 teaspoon paprika
- Oregano one fourth teaspoon
- Cumin ground one fourth teaspoon

Method

Take coconut flour, almond flour, psyllium husk, margarine, and salt in a bowl and mix well. Do it with your hands to make a crumbly dough (in a food processor, you can do that too). Add the water and knead over a little bit. The dough may appear a bit too wet, but as the flour absorbs the water, it will firm up. Divide the dough into eight tiny balls and put them in the fridge for ten minutes to rest.

Place the tvp in a small pot and add water until almost filled. Add the spices and the soya sauce. Boil it until the water is absorbed for about five minutes. Add the tomato sauce and allow it to cool down.

Set the temperature of your oven to 350 Fahrenheit. Take the dough from the refrigerator and roll it out into round disks of 2 mm (a little less than 1/8 inch), using a cut open zip lock bag to prevent it from sticking. If you have a press of tortilla, this is a good time to use it.

Take a spoon full of filling when you have rolled out the dough and fill it in the center. Fold over the plastic to form the empanada and close it.

If the dough breaks, simply gently rubbing the plastic with your fingers smooth out the cracks. Carefully take out the plastic from the formed empanada and put it on a parchment paper-lined baking sheet.

Bake the empanadas 12 minutes.

4.8 Smoked Maple Tempeh

Yield: 3 servings

Calories per serving: 195

Fat per serving: 12.7g

Carbs per serving: 3.4g net

Protein per serving: 15.8g

Fiber per serving: 4.6g

Salty, sweet, Smokey, and delicious, this easy dinner option is low carb and loaded with complete protein!

Ingredients

- Maple syrup sugar-free two tablespoons
- olive oil one tablespoon

- Tempeh one block eight grams
- Tamari low sodium one tablespoon

- olive oil one tablespoon

- Smoked half teaspoon

Method

Place the parchment lining paper on the baking sheet and preheat your oven to 350 F.

Whisk together in a bowl tamari, olive oil, sugar-free syrup, and salt, and set aside for a few minutes, so the flavors mix together, and the salt dissolves.

Cut the tempeh into pieces about one-fourth thick. Dip all the pieces of tempeh into the mixture so that it's totally covered, and place onto the baking sheet. Pour the remaining sauce over the tempeh and place the baking tray in the oven and bake for 30 minutes.

4.9 Roasted Bok Choy & Teriyaki Cauliflower Steaks

Preparation time: 10 minutes

Cooking time: 20 Minutes

Total time: 30 Minutes

Ingredients

- One tsp Garlic Powder

- Four Baby Bok Choy stalks

- Toasted Sesame Seeds half cup plus more

- Half Head Cauliflower, sliced into steaks

- Soy Sauce one cup

- Sesame Oil half cup, plus more to drizzle on Bok Choy

- Swerve Brown, two tablespoons

- Half tablespoon Ginger, paste or fresh

- Onion Powder one teaspoon

Method

Set oven temperature to 400. Whisk the dry and wet ingredients together and cook at medium heat to make the teriyaki sauce, and bring to a simmer. Reduce heat to low, and irregularly stir until sauce starts to thicken. Put the vegetables aside and chop them.

Wash bok choy leaves thoroughly and slices in half, lengthwise, per stalk. Sprinkle with sesame oil and sprinkle with salt to ensure each leaf is lightly coated. Dip the cauliflower steaks in the sauce and arrange on the sheet of cookies—roast for ten minutes.

Place the bok choy to the roasting pan and put it again in the oven for ten to fifteen minutes to the oven. Add sesame seeds to garnish.

4.10 Coconut Lime Noodles with Chili Tamari Tofu

Ingredients

For the Noodles

- Shirataki noodles two packs

- coconut milk one can

- One-fourth teaspoon red pepper flakes

- pinch of salt

For the Tofu

- One block (13.5oz/397g) extra firm tofu

- low sodium tamari four tablespoons

- olive oil one tablespoon

- one fourth tsp cayenne pepper

- Fresh grated ginger or ground half teaspoon
- sesame seeds four tablespoons
- juice and zest of 1 lime

Method

Drain and press out excess moisture of the tofu. Cut into roughly 1"x1" blocks.

Mix together olive oil, tamari, and cayenne. In a dish, place the tofu pieces in a single layer, and pour the mixture over the tofu. You'll have to flip the pieces a few times so that they are evenly covered. Heat your oven to 350 F, Place the tofu pieces on a baking sheet and bake for twenty minutes.

When the tofu is baking, risen and drain the noodles. Add to a frying pan on medium heat, along with the rest of the noodle ingredients and mix until well combined. Partially cover and cook for about ten minutes, then reduce the heat and continue cooking for another ten minutes.

Once the tofu is done, turn off the heat under the noodles as well. Then let everything cool for a few minutes before taking out in the dish. Garnish with lime zest, red pepper flakes, and sesame seeds.

4.11 Tofu and Bok Choy Salad

Ingredients

Oven-Baked Tofu

- 15 ounces extra-firm tofu
- One tablespoon sesame oil
- One tablespoon soy sauce
- One tablespoon water
- Two teaspoons minced garlic
- One tablespoon rice wine vinegar
- Juice ½ lemon

Bok Choy Salad

- Three tablespoons coconut oil
- Seven drops liquid stevia
- Nine ounces bok choy
- One stalk green onion
- Two tablespoons chopped cilantro
- Two tablespoons soy sauce
- One tablespoon sambal Olek
- One tablespoon peanut butter
- Half lime juice

Method

Press dry tofu, around 5-6 hours. Mix all the marinade ingredients sugar, soy sauce, sesame oil, garlic, lemon, and vinegar.

Chop the tofu into squares and put together with marinade in a plastic bag. Let this take at least thirty minutes to marinate, but ideally overnight.

Preheat the oven until 350F. Place tofu on a parchment paper-lined baking tray and bake for 35 minutes.

In a cup, mix all the salad dressing ingredients (except bok choy) together. Add cilantro and onion.

Chop the bok choy into tiny slices, much like the cabbage.

Remove the tofu from the oven, and add tofu, bok choy and sauce to your salad. Enjoy it!

4.12 Pumpkin Risotto

Serving Size: 1/4 batch

Calories per serving: 127

Fat per serving: 7.5g

Carbs per serving: 5.5g net

Protein per serving: 6.6g

Fiber per serving: 5.4g

Ingredients

- olive oil two tablespoons
- sliced leek one fourth cup
- paprika one teaspoon
- cauliflower riced three cups
- Pumpkin puree a half cup
- nutritional yeast one fourth cup
- veggie broth one-fourth cup or nondairy milk
- parsley fresh chopped one fourth cup
- salt and pepper to taste

Method

Add the olive oil, paprika, leek, salt, and pepper in a relatively large saucepan over medium heat.

Let the leek soften, irregularly stirring (cook until it's pretty translucent).

Add cauliflower, then stir until well mixed. Pour in the veggie broth and put the lid on the pan and let it cook for around fifteen minutes, stirring periodically so that the cauliflower stick is not present. Then add in nutritional yeast and pumpkin puree.

Taste the mixture (beware!)-if necessary, add more salt/pepper. If the cauliflower is still a little tough, cook until it becomes softer and more like rice.

Remove from heat the mixture, and garnish with parsley.

4.13 Halloumi with Strawberry and Cucumber Salsa

Preparation time: 10 minutes

Total time: 15 minutes

Protein20.8 grams

Net carbs6.8 grams

Calories449 kcal

Ingredients

- strawberries one cup
- jalapeño pepper one
- Cucumber half
- Lime juice one
- garlic clove minced one
- mint one tablespoon chopped
- basil chopped two tablespoons
- Olive oil extra virgin two tablespoons
- Halloumi cheese two packs
- balsamic vinegar one tablespoon
- Coconut butter one tablespoon
- pepper and salt to taste

Method

Peel the cucumber and dice. Dice the strawberries, jalapeno.

Wash and cut the herbs, mince garlic and combine along with the extra virgin olive oil, balsamic vinegar, and fresh lime juice. Mix everything in a bowl, sprinkle salt and pepper, and set aside. Slice the Halloumi cheese into half-inch slices and cook on both sides with ghee or butter. Cook both sides for two minutes or till crispy. Place on a serving plate and top with the strawberry & cucumber salsa.

4.14 Cheese-Stuffed Portobello Mushrooms

Protein14.3 grams

Net carbs5.5 grams

Fat28.5 grams

Calories334 kcal

Ingredients

- crumbled cheese one cup

- salt to taste

- Portobello mushrooms four

- fresh thyme

- lettuce (two cups

- Olive oil extra virgin two tablespoons

Method

Set the temperature of the oven to 350 ° F/175 ° C .Cut the mushrooms. Chop the stems in small pieces add thyme. Fill each mushroom with crumbled blue cheese, chopped stems, and thyme. Place in the oven for about twenty-five minutes. Remove from the oven and put fresh greens tossed with olive oil on a serving platter.

4.15 Bell Pepper Nachos

Preparation time: 15 minutes

Total time: 40 minutes

Ingredients

- Ground cumin half teaspoon
- Chili powder half teaspoon
- Kosher salt
- Lime wedges, for serving
- Bell peppers four
- Half pickled jalapeño slices
- One c. guacamole
- Olive oil extra virgin two tablespoons
- Garlic powder one fourth teaspoon
- Freshly ground black pepper
- One and a half c. shredded Monterey Jack
- One and a half shredded cheddar
- One Pico de Gallo salsa
- Half sour cream
- Milk or water one tablespoon

Method

Set the temperature of your oven to 425degrees, and line two small foil-based baking sheets.

Divide bell peppers for baking. Add olive oil, cumin, chili powder, and garlic powder to taste—season with salt and pepper. Place the wedges into a single layer on the baking sheets. Bake for about 10 minutes, until the peppers are crisp-tender. Top with Monterey Jack and cheddar. Bake for ten minutes. Top with guacamole, salsa, and jalapeños pickled. Put milk and sour cream together in a bowl, and chop over bell peppers. Squeeze on top of a lime wedge and serve with more lime wedges.

4.16 Spiralizer Zucchini Salad

Preparation time: 10 mins

Total time: 10 mins

Ingredients

- cabbage shredded one medium
- sunflower seeds shelled one cup
- zucchini thinly spiralizer one medium
- white vinegar cider vinegar one third cup

Stevia liquid one teaspoon

- almonds one cup sliced
- avocado oil three fourth cup

Method

Cut the spiralizer zucchini with the knife into smaller pieces.

Combine chives, sunflower seeds, and almonds in a bowl.

Put in the zucchini. Combine the oil, vinegar, and stevia in a small bowl and mix with a fork. Pour dressing on the mixture.

Chill for a total of 2 hours before serving to the optimum taste.

4.17 Low Carb Vegan Buddha Bowl

Preparation time: 10 minutes

Cooking time: 35 minutes

Total time: 45 minutes

Yield: 1 serving

Ingredients

- Broccoli florets one and a half cup
- Tahini two tablespoons

- Sesame seeds,
- Brussels sprouts one cup
- Oil half teaspoon
- Pumpkin seeds two tablespoons
- Avocado half
- Pinch of salt
- Kalamata olives ten

Method

Set oven temperature to 220 ° C (425 ° F). Add broccoli, Brussels sprouts, and pumpkin seeds, oil, tahini, and salt. Roast them for 35 minutes. Remove from the oven, whisk in Kalamata olives, and shake.

Serve in a dish with sliced avocado, and sprinkle with sesame seeds!

4.18 Peanut Butter Ramen

Preparation time: 10 minutes

Cooking time: 5 minutes

Total time: 15 minutes

Servings1

Calories574kcal

Ingredients

Sweet and Spicy Peanut Sauce

- sambal oelek one fourth cup

- soy sauce one and a half tablespoon

- Peanut butter one fourth cup

- sugar-free sweetener one teaspoon

Noodles and Toppings

- firm tofu one block

- Sesame seeds
- Shirataki noodles one pack
- Coconut oil one tablespoon
- Green onion chopped one or two
- Cayenne chili one chopped

Method

Cut the tofu into cubes and heat a medium-high skillet. Stir in the coconut oil (1 tbsp) and tofu. Stir so the tofu won't stick. Once the tofu starts browning, add soy sauce. Turn off the fire and set aside. You want to have a crispy outside the tofu.

Boil some water (a couple of cups will do). While the water boils, put the peanut butter with the sambal oelek (chili paste), soy sauce, and Truvia in a large bowl.

Slowly add 1/3 cup of the boiled water to the large bowl. Mix well to emulsify. Add more hot water, or less, depending on how liquid your peanut butter is.

Remove and strain the noodles from the package, and microwave for 2 minutes. Add the peanut sauce with the noodles and blend well. Once combined, transfer crispy tofu, sesame seeds, soy sauce, and chopped pepper to your bowl and top. Enjoy!

Chapter 5: Snacks Recipes

5.1 Tasty Avocado Fries

Serves: 1

Ingredients

- One-fourth cup of almond milk
- One avocado ripe
- Half cup almond flour
- Pepper, salt, and other spices to taste.

Method

Preheat your oven to 425F.

Place a parchment paper on the baking sheet.

Now peel your avocados and cut them in the shape of fries. Another easy way is to cut eight pieces from one avocado.

Now dip the pieces of avocado in milk and then in almond flour, sprinkle the spices, and then place those on the baking sheet.

Bake them for ten minutes, then turn the side and bake the other sides for ten minutes.

Take out from the oven and serve with chipotle hummus or any of your favorite sauce.

5.2 Mung Bean and Olive balls

Preparation time: 20 minutes

Cooking time: 25 minutes

Total time: 45 minutes

Serves: 4

Ingredients

- One tbsp. ground flaxseed
- One and a half cups mung beans cooked
- Half cup California black olives, finely chopped
- Half cup white onion, chopped
- One-fourth cup fresh parsley, chopped
- One-fourth tsp red chili flakes
- Two tablespoons tomato sauce, no sugar added.
- One garlic clove, minced
- Two tbsp. sun-dried tomatoes, chopped
- One tsp oregano dried
- One-fourth tsp freshly ground black pepper
- One fourth tsp salt

Instructions

Preheat your oven to 350°F.

Mix flaxseed with three tablespoons of water in a small bowl and set aside for at ten minutes.

Mash the beans with a food processor, potato masher or with a fork until a smooth texture forms in a medium bowl. Add olives, garlic, parsley, onion, tomatoes, spices, and tomato sauce.

When your flax egg has gelled, add it to the mixture too.

Roll the mixture into one and a half-inch balls and space evenly on a parchment paper placed on the baking sheet.

Cook for twenty minutes, take out from the oven, flip, and cook for five to ten minutes. When the balls turn brown, they are ready.

Serve the balls cold or warm over pasta or vegetables (Chelsey, 2020).

5.3 Chocolate Flourless Cookies

These flourless chocolate cookies made with almond flour/meal are your delicious snacks- fluffy, chewy, and made from only four ingredients! Of course, low carb, paleo, free of grain, and a tested vegan option! Gluten-Free, dairy-Free, refined Sugar-Free. Contrary to popular belief, a flax egg, which tends to be the most popular option, will not be used. You're going to use ground chia seeds instead of eggs. The end results will not be the same as those that use eggs, and it will be a little denser and crumbly.

Making these cookies extra high in protein

Although these cookies are naturally higher in protein than regular cookies, adding protein powder may allow you to go one step further.

The protein powder is 100% optional-Without; it works perfectly well.

Preparation time: 4 minutes

Cooking time: 10 minutes

Total time to cook: 14 minutes

Servings: 21cookies

Calories: 105kcal

Ingredients

- One cup almond flour
- Two tablespoons of chocolate protein powder optional
- One cup chocolate nut /seed butter of choice homemade or store-bought
- ground chia seeds
- One fourth cup chocolate chips

Instructions

Set the temperature of the oven to 350 degrees F and line a parchment paper on the baking tray or a silicone baking sheet.

Ina large bowl mix together all the ingredients or use mixer and mix until fully combined.

Form the cookie dough into small balls of golf size using your hands. Place onto the sheet of lined cookie or baking sheet. Use the palm of your hands and press lightly- Do not press into a whole shape of a cookie so that it remains quite thick.

Bake for 10-12 minutes, until just the edges are cooked. Take it out from the oven and place aside to cool for twenty minutes before being transferred to a wire rack and rest to cool.

3-4 tablespoons of ground chia seed for the vegan / egg-free version-Start with three tablespoons and increase to 4 if it is too thin

Cookies can be kept up to a week in a sealed jar. They taste well when refrigerated and last for two weeks. They are friendly to freezers, too.

5.4 Coconut Macaroons

Quick and simple no-bake coconut macaroons recipe- Only four ingredients and ready in ten minutes, these coconut macaroons are delicious low carb snacks. Gluten-Free, Vegan, and Paleo.

Preparation time: 5 minutes

Cooking time: 5 minutes

Total time: 10 minutes

Servings: 39 macaroons

Calories: 40kcal

Ingredients

- Coconut milk one fourth cup

- Shredded coconut unsweetened three cups

- Maple syrup keto three fourth cup

- Almond flour one cup

- Chocolate chips one cup

Instructions

- Place a parchment sheet on your baking tray and place it aside.

- Take a blender or a large mixing bowl and add all the ingredients in it and blend them well.

- If you find the batter crumbly, then add more coconut milk or sweetener to make a thick batter.

- Make small balls of the batter using your hands and then refrigerate them.

Monk fruit maple syrup, Maple syrup, agave, or brown rice syrup all work.

5.5 Pumpkin Spice Mousse

Preparation time: 10 minutes

Ingredients

- Pumpkin puree a half cup

- cashews soaked and drained one cup

- Maca optional one scoop

- Vanilla one teaspoon

- cashews soaked and drained one cup

- Pumpkin pie spice one teaspoon

- Cashew or almond butter two tablespoon

- Half+ more vegan milk of choice

Instructions

1. Soak cashews overnight and drain them.

2. Put all ingredients into a blender. Add a little milk then you think you will need.

3. for a thick and creamy texture add milk

4. Top with whipped cream (vegan). Keep it in the refrigerator.

5.6 Tortilla Chips

Preparation time: 5 mins

Cooking time: 14 mins

Total Time: 19 mins

Ingredients

- Tortillas low carb six

- Sea salt optional

- Olive oil or avocado oil

Instructions

- Preheat your oven to 350°F.

- Cut small triangles of tortillas.

- Spray oil on the baking tray and put the tortilla triangles on the tray.

- Spray more oil on the tortilla triangles and bake for seven minutes.

5.7 Almond Flour Crackers

Preparation time: 10 minutes

Cooking time: 15 minutes

Total time: 25 minutes

Ingredients

- Sunflower seeds two tablespoons
- Almond flour one cup
- Sea salt to taste
- Water two tablespoons
- Flax meal or whole psyllium husk one tablespoon
- One tablespoon coconut oil

Method

Preheat oven to 350 degrees F.

In a food processor or a bowl, add the almond flour, sunflower seeds, psyllium, and sea salt — finely chopped sunflower seeds. Blend them in a food processor.

Add in water and coconut oil until the dough forms when using a food processor. Stir the liquid ingredients into dry ingredients when blended by hand to form a dough.

Place the dough ball on a parchment paper sheet and press flat. Cover with another sheet of parchment paper and roll dough to a thickness of about 1/8 to 1/16 in.

Put on cutting board, remove the top parchment paper, and use a pizza cutter or knife to cut into 1-inch squares. If necessary, sprinkle with sea salt on top.

Place the cut dough on a baking sheet and bake at 350 ° F to brown and crisp edges (about 10-15 minutes). Let it cool on a rack and then divide it into squares.

5.8 Tamari Flax Crackers

These simple and easy low carb Tamari Seaweed Flax Crackers are flavorful and healthy! They are satisfying snacks.

Preparation time: 5 minutes

Dehydrate one day: 4 hour

Total time: 5 minutes

Servings: 30 crackers

Calories: 30kcal

Ingredients

- Flaxseeds golden half cup
- Flaxseeds half cup
- Water one and a half cup
- Tamari low sodium gluten-free two tablespoons
- Nori sheets two broken up (1/2 cup)

Directions

Soak the tamari and flaxseeds for at least one hour in water. Then add nori mix carefully.

Spoon 1 heap tablespoonful on a sheet of Teflon per cracker. Put in the dehydrator and dehydrate for 24-28 hours at 110 ° C, or until crispy. Turn over halfway through the dehydration process, and they dehydrate more rapidly.

5.9 Keto Vegan Chocolate Doughnuts

Preparation time: 5 minutes

Cooking time: 25 minutes

Total time: 30 minutes

Yield: 6

Serving Size: 1 doughnut

Calories per serving: 154

Fat per serving: 13g

Carbs per serving: 1.5g net

Protein per serving: 4.5g

Fiber per serving: 4.7g

Ingredients

Dry Ingredients

- Salt a pinch
- Baking powder half teaspoon
- Psyllium husk three tablespoons
- Cocoa powder three tablespoons

Wet Ingredients:

- Tahini half cup
- Granulated sweetener three tablespoons
- Brewed coffee or non-dairy milk of choice half cup
- Vanilla extract one teaspoon

Method

Preheat your oven to 177 ° C (350 ° F) and have a regular greased doughnut tray on hand.

Take a medium bowl, mix the dry ingredients together, and place them aside.

Mix all the wet ingredients together in a medium mixing bowl and keep mixing until everything is completely mixed.

Add all the ingredients dry and wet and mix them until they form a thick batter. Let this sit for five minutes so that the batter has time to thicken.

Distribute batter evenly into the doughnut pan and bake for 25 minutes, until the tops round the edges are firm and light brown. Remove from the oven and allow the doughnuts to cool for about 10 minutes before serving.

5.10 Pumpkin Stuffed Mushrooms

Preparation time: 10 minutes

Cooking time: 30 minutes

Total time: 40 minutes

Yield: 5

Calories per serving: 175

Fat per serving: 13.6g

Carbs per serving: 6g net

Protein per serving: 7.2g

Fiber per serving: 4.2g

Ingredients

- Nutritional yeast two tablespoons
- Walnuts one cup chopped
- Pumpkin half cup
- Mushroom caps six
- Flax seeds two tablespoons
- Salt half teaspoon
- onion powder half teaspoon
- garlic powder half teaspoon
- paprika half teaspoon
- ground black pepper, to taste

Method

Preheat your oven to 350F degrees.

Prepare mushrooms by cutting stems and gills, and clear any debris or soil. Place the stems aside.

Chop the mushroom stems thinly, and one of the caps.

Mix the spices, salt, flax seeds, and nutritional yeast together. In a medium-sized bowl, add pumpkin into the spice mixture, and mix until thoroughly mixed. Add the walnuts and finely chopped mushrooms, then mix until even.

Divide the filling into the remaining five mushroom caps and portion out.

Bake them for thirty minutes, or until the caps shrink in size, and all are tender

5.11 Keto Pie Crust

Preparation time: 5 minutes

Total time: 5 minutes

Yield: a single, 9-inch pie crust

Serving Size: 1/8 crust

Calories per serving: 150

Carbs per serving: 2.5g net

Fat per serving: 14g

Protein per serving: 4.6g

Fiber per serving: 6g

Ingredients

- Flax eggs two
- Coconut flour three fourth cup
- chilled, salted butter eight tablespoons

Method

Use a pastry cutter (or fork) in a mixing bowl to mix the coconut flour and butter until the texture is sandy, and no large butter lumps or floating dry pieces of coconut flour are present.

Add in two flax eggs, and mix until it forms a thick dough and can form into a ball.

If you find the dough too dry and crumbly here, you can add a tablespoon of cold water and keep kneading gently until the dough gets together.

Press the dough into a pie pan of 9

The crust is ready to be used in any recipe

5.12 Pumpkin Curry Crackers

Category: snack

Yield: 10 servings

Serving Size: ~1 ounce

Calories per serving: 177

Carbs per serving: 2.2g net

Fiber per serving: 8.1g

Fat per serving: 13.6g

Protein per serving: 6.7g

Ingredients

- pumpkin puree one cup
- cumin ground one teaspoon
- pumpkin seeds half cup
- curry powder one teaspoon
- flaxseeds, ground one, and a half cup

- salt one teaspoon

- ground black pepper one fourth teaspoon

Method

Set the oven temperature to 350 F and preheat it. And line a sheet of cookies with either parchment paper or a baking mat of silicon.

Mix together cumin, ground flax seeds, salt, curry powder, pepper, and pumpkin seeds in a mixing bowl until all is mixed.

Add the pureed pumpkin and blend until well blended. Let sit for a couple of minutes, so the flax absorbs the pumpkin all over.

Spread over the entire cookie sheet in a thin layer-it should be no more than 1/8 thick. Make sure that it is even; otherwise, the crackers will not cook properly.

Bake for forty-five minutes, test for doneness at forty minutes and go from there. The time will depend on how evenly your oven cooks, how moist the canned pumpkin was, and how thick the crackers are.

Take out from the oven once finished and allow it to cool for 10 minutes before breaking apart.

Let them cool and then store it in an airtight container. Theoretically, they should last like this for at least a week, but I have never eaten them all before.

5.13 Pancakes

Yield: 4-6 pancakes

Calories per serving: 220

Carbs per serving: 4g net

Fiber per serving: 11.5g

Fat per serving: 10.5g

Protein per serving: 17g

Ingredients

- Coconut flour one fourth cup

- Water one cup

- Psyllium husk two tablespoons soaked in half cup water

- vanilla one teaspoon

- protein powder one scoop

- Coconut oil one tablespoon

- baking powder one teaspoon

Method

In soaked psyllium husk, add in vanilla and coconut oil and place aside.

Mix all the dry ingredients together; Heat up a non-stick pan to medium pressure. Slowly add water in the dry ingredients and mix well.

Add psyllium mixture into protein powder mixture and stir until completely mixed. Batter Scoop onto the hot pan and spread it and heat for about five minutes, and flip over. Cook another five minutes on the other side.

5.14 Spice Blondies

Serving Size: 1 blondie

Calories per serving: 79

Carbs per serving: 1.8g net

Fiber per serving: 2.5g

Protein per serving: 3.2g

Ingredients

- Coconut flour one fourth cup

- pumpkin puree one cup

- Tahini half cup

- granulated sweetener or lakanto one fourth cup

- vanilla extract one teaspoon

- pumpkin pie spice one tablespoon

- apple cider vinegar one tablespoon

- baking powder one teaspoon

Method

Set the temperature of your oven to 350F and grease an eight square pan (if using a silicone pan! no greasing is required).

Mix pumpkin, tahini, sweetener, vanilla, and apple cider vinegar together.

Mix the coconut flour, spices, and baking powder together in a separate dish. Make sure everything is distributed properly. Add the wet mixture into dry ingredients and stir for about a minute to make sure everything is evenly mixed. Add into the brownie pan, and spread evenly and bake for 40 minutes.

5.15 Peanut Butter Chocolate Milkshake

Calories79kcal

Ingredients

- unsweetened cocoa powder one tablespoon

- Peanut butter powder unsweetened one tablespoon

- coconut milk unsweetened one cup

- Stevia drops five

Method

Blend them all in the blender until mix well.

5.16 Spinach smoothie

Preparation time: 5 minutes

Total time: 5 minutes

Yield: 1 Smoothie

Ingredients

- Matcha powder half teaspoon
- Vanilla extract one teaspoon
- spinach blend two-third cup
- avocado medium half
- Golden monk fruit sweetener one tablespoon
- coconut milk half cup
- water two-third cup
- Ice
- MCT oil powder one scoop

Optional additions:

- Vanilla protein powder one fourth cup
- Chia seeds half tablespoon

Instructions

Put all the above-mentioned ingredients to a blender and blend until mixed well.

5.17 Peanut Butter Chocolate Fudge

Preparation time: 5 minutes

Cooking time: 1 hour

Total time: 1 hour 5 minutes

Ingredients

- Peanut Butter one fourth cup

- Stevia one fourth cup

- Dark Chocolate 100 grams

Directions

In a pan, placed the dark chocolate, peanut butter, and stevia.

Heat up over low heat until the chocolate has melted completely.

Turn off the heat once the chocolate has melted.

Prepare a small rectangular dish greased it and add the melted chocolate and peanut butter. Place in the fridge to prepare for a few hours.

Remove from the refrigerator and cut into bits of fudge.

5.18 Baked Tofu

Ingredients

- Firm tofu one block

- Cornstarch one tablespoon

- Liquid aminos one fourth cup

Method

Drain tofu: remove tofu from the box, and wrap tofu block in towels of paper. Squeeze the excess moisture gently, and set aside for about 10 minutes to allow it to continue to drain.

Preheat oven to 425F. When the tofu has been drained, cut into cubes and put into a large mixing bowl. Pour liquid aminos and sprinkle the cornstarch over tofu and toss until coated evenly, and there is no visible dry cornstarch. Place the pieces of tofu on the baking sheet and bake 30 minutes.

5.19 Peanut Butter Sauce

Ingredients

- Peanut flour protein plus one fourth cup
- Soy sauce low sodium two tablespoons
- Ginger one teaspoon
- Lakanto Monk fruit sweetener six drops
- Garlic powder half teaspoon
- Water two tablespoon
- Lime juice one tablespoon

Method

Take all the ingredients and mix them in a bowl

Chapter 6: Dinner Recipes

6.1 Pesto Zucchini Zoodles

Preparation time: 10 minutes

Cooking time: 10 mins

Total time: 20 mins

Course: Dinner

Servings: Three persons

Calories: 226 kcal

Ingredients

- Two medium zucchini, spiralizer
- One third cup vegan pesto plus more if needed
- Six mushrooms, thinly sliced
- Ten cherry tomatoes, cut from the center
- Two cloves garlic, finely minced
- Two teaspoon olive oil
- Half red onion, thinly sliced and halved
- salt, to taste
- Black pepper grounded
- Crushed red pepper
- Two cloves garlic, finely minced
- cashew cream for drizzle

Directions

In a nonstick pan, heat the olive oil over medium to high heat.

Add sliced onions, chopped garlic, and sliced chickpeas.

Add one fourth teaspoon salt.

Stir fry the vegetables until tender, but still remain crispy. The water released from cooking mushrooms should be dried.

Quickly wipe a wet napkin over the pan.

Heat one fourth cup pesto, add the spiralizer zucchini spaghetti, and sauté for 1-2 minutes on medium-high heat to cook easy.

Add the cherry tomato halves and the sautéed onions/mushrooms.

Bring the rest of the pesto in. If necessary, please feel free to add more pesto than the amount given above.

(Optional) Add a cashew cream drizzle, if you want.

Sauté, tossing regularly for another 1-2 minutes.

Add some salt to taste, freshly ground black pepper, and crushed red pepper (if used).

Serve cold or warm, enjoy! Keep the remains in the fridge in an airtight jar (Lalani, 2017).

6.2 Walnut Chili

This vegan keto walnut chili is a simple and delicious Gluten-Free, Low Carb High Protein dinner recipe.

Preparation time: 10 minutes

Cooking time: 31 minutes

Total time: 41 minutes

Course: Dinner

Servings: seven persons

Ingredients

- Two tablespoons of olive oil extra virgin

- Two cloves garlic minced
- Five stalks celery finely diced
- One and a half teaspoon of cinnamon grounded
- Two teaspoon chili powder
- Four teaspoon cumin ground
- One and a half tsp smoked paprika
- Two peppers large chipotle in adobo minced
- Two green bell peppers finely diced
- Two zucchini diced
- Eight oz. cremini mushrooms minced
- One and a half tablespoon tomato sauce
- Half cup of coconut milk
- 1 15 oz. can diced tomatoes
- Three cups of water
- Add pepper and salt according to your taste
- two and a half cups soy meat crumbled
- One cup walnuts minced
- One tablespoon unsweetened cocoa powder

For serving

- One avocado sliced
- Two tablespoon fresh cilantro leaves
- Two tbsp. Sliced radishes

Method

- On medium flame heat oil in a large pan.
- Add the celery and cook for four minutes, then add in the garlic, chili powder, paprika, cumin, cinnamon, and

paprika and fry them until fragrant, about two more minutes.

- Add the zucchini, bell peppers, mushrooms, and cook for about five minutes.

- Add the tomatoes, walnuts, cocoa powder, water, tomato paste, coconut milk, soy meat, and chipotle.

- Lower the heat to medium to low flame and simmer for about 25 minutes until it becomes thick and the vegetables become soft.

- Sprinkle with pepper and salt to taste. Top with radish avocado and cilantro (Sharp, 2018).

6.3 Lo Mein

Category: Dinner

Yield: 1 large lo mein bowl

Serving Size: one person

195 Calories per serving

Fat: 13.9 g per serving

Carbs per serving: net 4.4 g

Protein: 5.1 g

Fiber on each serving: 4.5 g

This gluten-free, low-carb vegan lo mein is a great replacement to a classic take-out. Making it easy, delicious, and keto-friendly!

Ingredients

Shirataki noodles one pack (drained and rinsed)

Broccoli one cup

Carrots shredded two tablespoon

The sauce

- Tamari two tablespoons
- One tablespoon sesame oil
- Garlic minced half teaspoon
- One fourth tsp Sriracha (or whatever peppery chili sauce you might have!)

Directions

Open shirataki noodles, and add water in it.

Toss in sauce ingredients, as well as broccoli, in a saucepan at medium-low heat.

Once the pan has reached temp, put in the noodles and cover them (drain the water from the noodles before putting them in the oven).

Let it simmer for a couple of minutes, stirring the noodles to spread them, so they are soft and absorb the sauce. When the pan becomes hot, add a few tablespoons of water to keep things from burning and allow the sauce to cook.

When the noodles have softened, mix all together until the ingredients are well distributed, turn off the burner and let the noodles sit in the pan until all the liquid in the bottom is absorbed.

Serve, and then enjoy!

6.4 Lasagna Zucchini with Tofu Ricotta and Walnut Sauce

Preparation time: 10 minutes

Cooking time: 35 minutes

Total time: 45 minutes

Servings: four persons

Calories: 356kcal

Ingredients

Walnut Sauce

- 1 (25 ounces) jar marinara sauce, divided
- Walnuts one cup grounded.
- Tomatoes sun-dried chopped one fourth cup

Lasagna

- whole batch tofu
- Two zucchini
- Nutritional yeast two tablespoons

Method

Preheat the oven to 375 ° C. Mix the walnuts, marinara sauce, and sun-dried tomatoes.

1/16 "lengthwise slice of zucchini on a mandolin. Pour 3/4 cup marinara sauce into a 7 1/2 "x 9 1/2" pan. Add zucchini noodles on marinara sauce, overlapping each slice — Spread 1/3 of tofu over zucchini noodles. Sprinkle yeast on top of tofu. Pour half of the walnut sauce on top.

Layer more zucchini noodles, then 1/3 tofu, nutritional yeast, and rest walnut sauce. Complete with a layer of zucchini noodles, tofu ricotta, and nutritional yeast. Bake for 35 minutes at 375 ° C.

6.5 Hemp Seed Cauliflower Rice Pilaf

Preparation time: 5 minutes

Cooking time: 5 minutes

Total time: 10 minutes

Servings: Four

Course: Side dish

Calories: 224kcal

Ingredients

- Half head of cauliflower makes two cups cauliflower rice
- Hemp seeds half cup
- 1/2 teaspoon turmeric
- Vegetable broth low sodium half cup
- Salt and pepper
- Pitted dates Four chopped
- Turmeric half teaspoon
- cumin half teaspoon
- One-fourth cup sliced almonds

Directions

When using a cauliflower head, cut it into large chunks and place it inside the food processor. Mix until it resembles the consistency of rice.

Place cauliflower rice with hemp seeds, chopped dates, turmeric, cumin, vegetable broth and salt and pepper in a saucepan. Cook, for five minutes, until liquid is absorbed. Add almonds (Moon, 2017).

6.6 Pesto Shirataki Noodles

These low carb vegan keto pesto shirataki noodles are perfect for people on a keto vegan diet.

Preparation time: 5 minutes

Cooking time: 3 minutes

Total time: 8 minutes

Servings: Four persons

Calories: 190kcal

Ingredients

- One clove garlic minced
- pine nuts one fourth cup
- Nutritional yeast one fourth cup
- Shirataki noodles two packs
- Two cups packed fresh basil.
- Pistachio oil or olive oil one fourth cup
- pinch salt

Method

Drain and rinse the shirataki noodles thoroughly: boil three minutes, or one minute microwave.

Add the remaining ingredients in the blender add olive oil while the motor is on.

Mix the pesto and the shirataki noodles together and serve.

6.7 Bibimbap

An easy, delicious, and spicy gluten-free and low carb dinner recipe!

Serving Size: 1 bowl

Calories per serving: 247

Fat per serving: 12.7g

Carbs per serving: 9.5g net

Protein per serving: 18g

Fiber per serving: 8.7g

Ingredients

- cooked broccoli half cup

- Gochujang low carb one tablespoon

- sesame seeds one teaspoon

- cauliflower rice cooked one cup

- baked or air-fried tofu 3.5oz

- cooked shiitake mushrooms 1/8 cup

- Chopped scallions for garnish

Method

Reheat the cauliflower rice and veggies on the stove and bake for thirty minutes at 350 F or air-fry the tofu for twenty minutes or when it is crispy. Mix all vegetables and tofu together in a bowl, add in gochujang and garnish with scallions and sesame seeds.

Alternatively, arrange tofu and veggies in a dish top with scallions, gochujang, and sesame seeds, take pictures and then mix and eat

6.8 Broccoli Soap

Ingredients

- One onion, chopped
- Freshly ground pepper to taste
- 1/2 teaspoon salt
- Three cloves garlic, pressed
- Two tablespoons nutritional yeast flakes
- One tablespoon oil
- Broccoli one pound
- One large carrot, in chunks
- Turmeric half teaspoon
- Water 750 ml
- One vegan bouillon cube
- 100-gram unroasted cashews, boiled for 10 minutes or soaked for 2-4 hours

- 250 ml of water
- Two tablespoons miso
- Two tablespoons lemon juice

Method

Heat a big pan over medium flame and sauté the onion in the oil until it is soft and odorless. Add in the garlic and sauté for another half minute. Add and bring to a boil the broccoli, bouillon, carrot, turmeric, and 750 ml water. Cook until the carrots are tender, for about ten minutes.

Make the cashew sauce, meanwhile. Blend the soaked cashews in a blender to a completely smooth liquid along with the miso and nutritional yeast. This might take up to several minutes, depending on the strength of your machine.

When cooking, the vegetables puree the soup. It's good to give the broccoli and carrots a little texture, so don't make it too smooth. Add the sauce to the soup and give another ten minutes to simmer so it can thicken. Finally, add the juice of a lemon and the pepper. If you think it needs that, taste the soup and add a little more lemon juice, pepper, or salt. Serve it alone or with bread low in carb.

6.9 Crack Slaw

Ingredients

- green cabbage four cups shredded

- One teaspoon chili paste, kimchi paste (make sure it's vegan!), or sriracha

- sesame oil one tablespoon

- macadamia nuts, half cup chopped

- vinegar one teaspoon

- Liquid aminos or tamari two tablespoons

- garlic cloves two
- green onion and sesame seeds to garnish

Method

Toss cabbage in a saucepan at medium-low heat with vinegar, tamari, sesame oil, and /kimchi paste/chili paste/sriracha. Add in chopped garlic.

Cover the pan and sit for about five minutes, until the cabbage begins to soften. Mix it well in the pan, add nuts.

Cook for five or six minutes until some extra liquid in the pan is absorbed by the nuts. Serve, and enjoy.

6.10 Vegan Fathead Pizza Crust

Preparation time: 5 minutes

Cooking time: 30 minutes

Total time: 35 minutes

Category: dinner

Cuisine: vegan keto

Serving Size: 1/3 crust

Calories per serving: 223

Carbs per serving: 1.8g net

Fiber per serving: 11.7g

Fat per serving: 17.8g

Protein per serving: 6.6g

Ingredients

- vegan cream cheese one fourth cup
- Psyllium husk two tablespoons
- baking powder one teaspoon

*
*   ground flaxseed three fourth cup

*   salt half teaspoon

*   Garlic powder one teaspoon

*   water half cup

Method

Set the temperature of your oven to 350F and preheat it. Line with parchment paper or a baking mat with silicone.

Mix all of the dry ingredients together. Cut cream cheese and add water slowly to the mixture, mix thoroughly before adding more water.

Put dough on the baking mat when all the water is incorporated, and flatten into a quarter-inch-thick pizza shape. The quick and easy way to do this is by rolling the dough out between two parchment paper pieces! You can also flatten it by hand. Bake the round for fifteen minutes, then turn thoroughly and bake for another five minutes.

Remove from the oven, sprinkle the pesto, sauce, veggies. Bake for another 10-15 minutes (depending on toppings). Remove, just let it cool and enjoy!

6.11 Carbonara

Preparation time: 30 minutes

Cooking time: 10 minutes

Total time: 40 minutes

Calories per serving: 410

Carbs per serving: 2.4g net

Fiber per serving: 7.4g

Fat per serving: 28g

Protein per serving: 30g

Ingredients

For the Tofu (makes four servings)

- low-sodium tamari one block

- olive oil two tablespoons

- firm tofu one block

- Smoked sea salt one fourth teaspoon

For the sauce (makes five servings):

- Hemp seeds hulled one cup

- Nutritional yeast three fourth cup

- Salt one fourth teaspoon

- Water three fourth cup

For the Whole Dish:

- shirataki noodles one pack

- The above sauce one third cup

- Above mentioned tofu one fourth batch

- nutritional yeast one teaspoon

- scallion stalk sliced one

- Fresh black pepper

Set the temperature of the oven to 375 ° F and line a parchment paper rimmed baking sheet. Drain the tofu, and thinly slice it. Use a dishtowel to press the water out of the tofu slices.

Whisk together the tamari, olive oil and smoked sea salt in a small blending bowl.

In the marinade, dip each piece of tofu and place it on the baking sheet.

Garnish any remaining marinade over bits of tofu. Bake for thirty minutes, until it becomes crispy.

To Make Sauce:

Add all sauce ingredients to a food processor and blend them until totally smooth, about three minutes.

Drain and rinse the shirataki noodles and place them in a small pan on medium-low heat. Add one-third cup of the sauce to the noodles and stir until the noodles are thoroughly coated.

Cook for ten minutes until the sauce is thick, and the excess moisture cooks out of the noodles. Cut the slices of bacon and stir the pieces with the noodles.

Cover and sprinkle on additional nutritional yeast and fresh pepper, if desired.

6.12 Spinach and Ricotta Bake

Serving: 1

Calories: 402

Protein: 23.8g

Fat: 31.4g

Net Carbs: 8.9g

Preparation time: 15 mins

Cooking time: 40 mins

Total time: 55 mins

Ingredients

- garlic clove one chopped
- frozen spinach 600 grams
- Himalayan salt to taste
- Olive oil extra virgin 20 ml

- paprika
- organic broth granules sprinkle
- Flax eggs two
- Vegan cream 50 ml
- nutmeg
- black pepper to taste
- ricotta 250 grams
- Vegan cheese
- Parmesan 75 grams

Method

Sprinkle extra virgin olive oil over a shallow pan.

Add the ginger, spinach, broth granules, black pepper, nutmeg, and paprika.

Stir and cook until it's dry and just start crackling, then taste test and set aside to cool.

Preheat oven to fan 180c. Add in flax eggs until the volume tripled. Add the ricotta again, and mix. Add milk and mix again.

Add salt, a black pepper, cooled spinach and cheese

Mix it all up and put it into a 20 cm x 30 cm buttered oven dish.

Add the remaining cheese over the top, even with the back of a spoon.

Bake for thirty minutes when raising the oven to 200C and bake for another 8-10 minutes until golden brown on top.

6.13 Avocado Arugula Tomato Salad

Preparation time: 15 minutes

Total time: 15 minutes

Servings: Four

Calories: 269kcal

Ingredients

Tomato Salad -

- red cherry tomatoes, cut in half one pint
- Arugula, roughly chopped five oz.
- basil leaves, sliced thinly six large
- cherry or grape tomatoes Yellow one pint halved
- firm avocados two large
- red onion, diced none fourth cup

Balsamic Vinaigrette -

- Olive oil one tablespoon
- Balsamic vinegar two tablespoons
- Maple syrup one tablespoon
- Lemon juice one tablespoon
- garlic clove, minced one
- Pink sea salt one fourth teaspoon
- pepper one fourth teaspoon
- Italian seasoning half teaspoon

In a large mixing bowl, place the halved tomatoes, arugula, red onion, basil leaves, and avocado. Add the vinegar, maple syrup, olive oil, lemon juice, salt, garlic, Italian seasonings, and pepper in a small bowl until well blended. Pour over the tomato salad over the dressing. Mix the salad and add fresh basil to garnish.

6.14 Mashed Cauliflower, Herbs and Garlic

Preparation time: 10 minutes

Cooking time: 10 minutes

Total time: 20 minutes

Serving: 4 servings

Ingredients

- Olive oil one tablespoon
- Cauliflower one head
- Minced garlic cloves two
- chopped herbs, rosemary, thyme, parsley, chives, and sage

Method

Trim the cauliflower stems, and cut off the florets and wash them in water.

Heat 1-inch of water over medium heat in a pot, and bring to a boil. Add the florets of the cauliflower and steam them for 6-8 minutes.

While steaming the cauliflower, heat up the olive oil on medium heat in a small pan. Add the chopped garlic and cook for thirty seconds before removing from oil.

Remove the steamed cauliflower from the pot, drain the pot water, and then put it back in the pan. Stir in olive oil, onions, chopped herbs, and any other ingredients. Mash the cauliflower using a potato masher.

6.15 Balsamic-Glazed Mushrooms

Preparation time: 15 minutes

Cooking time: 2 hours

Total Time: 2 hours 15 minutes

Servings: Four Servings

Calories: 210kcal

Ingredients

- Garlic cloves chopped
- Maple syrup two tablespoons
- Tamari one tablespoon
- Mushrooms 32 ounces
- Olive oil extra virgin one fourth cup
- balsamic vinegar two tablespoons
- black pepper one fourth teaspoon
- sea salt half teaspoon

Method

Cut off stems tip of all the mushrooms. Clean all the mushrooms with a damp cloth. Add all the ingredients and mix them into a slow cooker.

Cook for 2 to 3 hours at high.

6.16 Pasta with Vegan Alfredo Sauce (high protein pasta)

Preparation time: 10 minutes

Cooking time: 10 minutes

Total Time: 20 minutes

Yield: 2 servings

Ingredients

- Italian style vegan sausages two
- spinach fettuccine noodles half box

For the Sauce

- onion half cup chopped
- tofu half cube
- rosemary one fourth teaspoon
- olive oil one teaspoon
- salt half teaspoon
- mustard one teaspoon
- garlic cloves four
- onion powder half teaspoon
- the black pepper one fourth teaspoon
- parsley one teaspoon
- Thyme one fourth teaspoon
- Water half cup
- vegan mayo one teaspoon
- nutritional yeast two tablespoons

Sauté the chopped onions over medium heat in a pan with around one tsp oil.

After they start softening, add the garlic and sauté for another couple of minutes until both are soft.

Turn off the fire. Combine the tofu, onions, and garlic in a food processor and blend until smooth. Apply the remaining sauce ingredients to the food processor, then blend until smooth and well mixed.

Cook pasta after reading to the instructions on the box.

Slice the vegan sausages and sauté each side for a few minutes over medium heat in the oven.

Pour the sauce to the pan and cook, stirring periodically, until warm through. Put the sauce over the pasta and serve immediately.

6.17 Roasted Peppers and Onions

Preparation time: 5 mins

Cooking time: 30 mins

Total time: 35 mins

Servings: Four

Ingredients

- orange bell pepper one
- red bell pepper one
- small onion one
- yellow bell pepper one
- smoked paprika half teaspoon
- oregano one fourth teaspoon
- salt pinch
- pepper pinch
- avocado oil one teaspoon

Directions

Preheat the oven until 400 degrees F.

Slice the onions and peppers. Place the sliced vegetables on a baking sheet and spray the foil and Bake for 20 minutes.

Chapter 7: Recipes for Kids

7.1 Oreo-Esque Protein Cookies (zero carbs)

Preparation time: 10 minutes

Cooking time: 5 to 6 minutes

Total time: 6 minutes

Ingredients for cookies

- Two tablespoon syrup IMO
- Two tablespoon chocolate or vanilla whey
- Four tablespoons black cocoa onyx powder

Filling Ingredients

- One tablespoon cheese mascarpone
- Vanilla whey protein: 1/8-1/4 cup

Method

First, make your cookies by tossing all the above-mentioned cookie ingredients in a bowl and combining them with a spoon until you get a soft dough that you can mold with your hands into 'balls' (it'll feel like play-dough!) If your dough is too sticky to allow you to do this, add a little more cocoa powder until you get the right consistency.

Shape 6-10 'balls' out of the mixture depending on how large you want your cookies and flatten them with your hands and put them on a non-stick baking tray or a regular cookie tray lined with baking paper.

Bake for no more than five minutes at 200C (approx. 395 F).

They normally take five minutes to cook so, please check them out after 5 minutes and take them out of the oven if cooked through.

Mix all of your ingredients together to make your filling. If you like your mix to be creamier than, then use casein!

Fill the filling into the cookies, and here your protein pack low carb cookies are ready.

Recommendations

- Use onyx to turn your cookies Oreo-like, but if you don't care about it, you can use normal use cocoa powder.
- You should then use the quark or cream cheese
- Depends on how thick your mix is

7.2 Eggless Chocolate Brownie

A moist, soft, fluffy and gooey brownie ready in minutes and surely low carb too! Made with no oil, sugar, or grains. This healthy single-serving mug brownie is vegan, paleo, and keto, gluten-free, dairy-free, sugar-free, and low calorie

Preparation time: 2 minutes

Cooking time: One minute

Total Time: Three minutes

Servings: One brownie

Calories: 196kca

Ingredients

- Cocoa powder one tablespoon
- Granulated sweetener one tablespoon
- Almond butter one tablespoon
- Baking powder one eight teaspoon
- almond milk or coconut milk three tablespoons
- Almond flour two tablespoons
- Chocolate chips one tablespoon

Method

- Take a microwave-safe ramekin or a bowl and grease it with oil spray.

- Add the dry ingredients in a bowl and mix them well.

Combine your smooth milk and almond butter and mix together in a separate bowl.

Mix all the dry and wet ingredients and mix them well. If adding chocolate chips, fold them through.

Place the bowl in the microwave for thirty seconds.

Take out the bowl and keep aside for one minute for cooling.

Instructions for oven

- For baking it in the oven, preheat your oven 180C/350F.

- Grease your baking dish and add the batter.

- Bake the brownie for six minutes.

- Take it out from the oven and set aside to cool for a minute, then slice and serve.

7.3 Pumpkin Chocolate Chip Cookies

Preparation time: 10 minutes

Cooking time: 18 minutes

Total time: 28 minutes

Yield: 18 cookies

Ingredients

- Almond flour two cups

- Half teaspoon stevia sweetener

- Baking powder half teaspoon

- Coconut oil one fourth cup
- Half cup almond butter
- Half cup of organic pumpkin puree
- Cinnamon one-fourth teaspoon
- 2 tablespoons of vegan cream cheese
- Two flax eggs (2 tablespoons of flax with six tablespoons of water)
- Himalayan salt a pinch
- Vanilla bean powder a pinch

Method

Heat the oven at 350 degrees. Mix two tablespoons of water with flax seeds grounded and leave it for ten to twenty minutes.

Except for chocolate chips) mix all the remaining ingredients well in a mixing bowl using your hand or a mixer.

Add chocolate chips in it and make the shape of cookies with your hand.

Bake the cookies for twenty minutes, then take them out from the oven leave for 5 minutes and serve.

7.4 Tofu Fries

Preparation time: 30 minutes

Cooking time: 40 minutes

Total time: 1 hour 10 minutes

Servings: Four people

Calories: 132kcal

Ingredients

- 1/4 teaspoon paprika
-

- 15.5 ounces tofu extra firm pressed and drained
- Two tablespoons olive oil
- basil half teaspoon
- One fourth teaspoon garlic powder
- One fourth teaspoon cayenne pepper
- Half teaspoon oregano
- onion powder one fourth teaspoon
- Salt and pepper

Directions

Preheat the oven until 375 ° C.

Mix all the herbs and spices and the olive oil.

Slice of tofu into long strips, around 1/4-1/2 wide.

Marinade the strips.

Place strips on a baking dish lined with parchment paper and bake at 375 ° for twenty minutes. Flip and bake for another twenty minutes or until the outside is crispy.

7.5 Coconut Peanut Butter Balls

Ingredients

- Coconut flakes unsweetened half cup
- peanut butter three tablespoons
- cocoa powder unsweetened three teaspoons
- powdered erythritol two and a half teaspoon
- almond flour two teaspoons

Method

Mix together in bowl cocoa, peanut butter, erythritol, and flour.

Freeze for an hour.

Using a small spoon, takeout a small serving of the peanut butter mix.

Put it into the coconut flakes and roll around with hands, so the coconut covers the ball. Shape them into a ball if needed. Keep them in the fridge overnight, so they firm up.

7.6 Chocolate Peppermint Chia Pudding

Preparation time: 10 minutes

Serving: Six

Calories: 126 KCAL

Ingredients

- Peppermint extract half teaspoon
- Himalayan salt three fourth teaspoon
- Almond milk or coconut milk sixty ml
- Cocoa powder 38grams
- Swerve or xylitol four to eight tablespoons
- unsweetened almond milk 475ml
- Chia seeds hundred grams

Method

Add all the ingredients to a wide bowl, beginning with four tablespoons sweetener, and blend until thoroughly mixed. Sweeten to taste and refrigerate until thickened (preferably!), three hours to overnight. Thin it out with more almond milk or water as required, if necessary, and according to taste.

If the whole texture isn't your thing, just mix it up until silky smooth! Or from the start, using powdered chia seeds.

Yeah, and just before serving, feel free to sprinkle it with the Himalayan pink salt, a perfect way to include this salt in your diet!

Keep this chocolate chia pudding in an airtight container, refrigerated for up to three days.

7.7 White Chocolate Raspberry Cups

Yield: 12 raspberry cups

Serving Size: 1 raspberry cup

Calories per serving: 158

Fat per serving: 15.5

Carbs per serving: 1g net

Protein per serving: 2.6g

Fiber per serving: 1.4g

Ingredients

- Coconut manna half cup
- Cocoa butter half cup
- Crushed dried freeze raspberries one fourth cup
- Coconut milk powder four tablespoons
- Swerve three tablespoons
- Vanilla extract one teaspoon

Method

Melt cacao butter and cacao manna in a double boiler and mix until thoroughly combined. Add vanilla extract and mix the coconut milk powder and the Swerve in a separate bowl.

Stir the whey / Swerve mixture one tablespoon at a time into the cacao butter/coconut manna, making sure it's thoroughly absorbed before adding the next spoon. Mix the dried raspberries in it.

Slice into a muffin tin. You can use the silicone to make your life easier.

Chill up for about an hour in the refrigerator before eating.

7.8 Pumpkin Spice Doughnuts

Preparation time: 5 minutes

Cooking time: 30 minutes

Total Time: 35 minutes

Yield: 12 mini doughnuts

Calories per serving: 44 (88)

Fat per serving: 3.2g (6.4g)

Carbs per serving: 1g net (2.2g)

Protein per serving: 1g (2g)

Fiber per serving: 1.8g (3.6g)

Ingredients

- Coconut flour one fourth cup
- Flax seeds grounded two tablespoons
- Pumpkin spice seasoning one tablespoon
- Vanilla extract one teaspoon
- Baking powder one teaspoon
- Coconut oil two tablespoons
- Non-dairy milk or water one fourth cup
- Canned pumpkin half cup

- Swerve two tablespoons

Method

Use a silicone doughnut pan or grease muffin tin with coconut oil.

Preheat oven to 350F. Add the water into the ground flax seeds, and let sit for a couple of minutes.

Add the canned pumpkin, Swerve, vanilla, and coconut oil to the flaxseed mixture.

Mix the dry ingredients cinnamon, coconut flour, baking powder, and spices together in a separate bowl.

Add the dry and wet ingredients and mix them well. Batter scoop into the doughnut pan holes.

Bake them for thirty minutes. The doughnuts are done, as they're going to separate a little bit from the sides of the tin.

Before removing from the pan, let it cool completely by inverting it on a cutting board.

7.9 Chocolate Almond Butter Pie

Yield: 12 slices of pie

Serving Size: 1/12th pie

Calories per serving: 359

Carbs per serving: 5.1g net

Fat per serving: 42.5g

Fiber per serving: 5.9g

Protein per serving: 6.5g

Ingredients

For the Crust:

- Coconut oil half cup

- Coconut flour three fourth cup

- Psyllium husk two tablespoon

- Water half cup

- salt a pinch

For the Filling

- Almond butter one cup

- Chocolate unsweetened thirty grams

- One can coconut milk

- coconut oil one fourth cup

- stevia (optional) one fourth teaspoon

Method

Oven preheats to 350F. Melt the water and coconut oil together in a bowl. Add in the husk of psyllium to make the gel. Mix the flour and salt in the coconut and let sit for a minute or two until all the liquid has been absorbed.

Push the crust into a 9 "pie dish. Try making the crust as thick as possible, so it bakes evenly.

Poke a fork at the bottom of the crust several times (it's called "docking," and it helps release air so that the crust doesn't puff up strangely) and bake for thirty minutes.

As the crust is baking, mix the remaining ingredients in a high-blender and process until they are thoroughly mixed. You may first melt the chocolate to make things easier.

Remove the crust from the oven and allow to cool for a few minutes before pouring in the filling. Place it in the fridge for seven hours or freeze it for three hours.

7.10 Red Velvet Cupcakes

Yield: 4 cupcakes

Serving Size: 1 cupcake

Calories per serving: 208

Carbs per serving: 4.6g net

Fiber per serving: 4.3g

Fat per serving: 19g

Protein per serving: 5.8g

Ingredients

For the Cupcakes

- Almond butter or tahini one fourth cup
- Non-dairy milk or unsweetened coconut milk one fourth cup
- Granulated sweetener two tablespoons
- Apple cider vinegar one tablespoon
- Flax seed grounded two tablespoons
- Cocoa powder two tablespoons
- Beetroot powder one tablespoon
- Baking powder half teaspoon
- Baking soda one fourth teaspoon

For the Frosting

- Coconut cream one fourth cup
- The vegan cream cheese one fourth cup
- Liquid stevia, to taste 4 to 5 drops

Method

Preheat the oven until 350F. Line 4 wells with a standard size muffin pan with paper liners or a standard size silicone muffin pan or muffin liners.

Mix the coconut, milk tahini, and vinegar together in a small mixing bowl until well blended and smooth. Add the sweetener and flax seeds.

Use a fork to whisk the beetroot powder, cocoa powder, baking powder, and baking soda together in a separate bowl until thoroughly mixed. Break any clumps with the fork.

Fold the dry ingredient into the wet and mix until no clumps remain. Be sure not to stir too roughly because you want to preserve some of the volume created by the reaction to baking soda and vinegar.

Divide the batter evenly between the four-lined muffin wells, each filling in about 3/4 of the way. Bake for thirty minutes.

Take them out from the oven and keep them aside to cool for at least ten minutes,

For frosting, mix the cream cheese and coconut cream (and optional stevia) together until smooth, then evenly divide into the cupcakes.

7.11 Peanut Clusters

Preparation time: 10 mins

Cooking time: 10 mins

Total time: 20 mins

 Calories69kcal

Ingredients

- Vanilla stevia drops a half teaspoon

- Coconut oil one tablespoon

- baking chocolate unsweetened four ounces

- Planters Cocktail peanuts six ounces

Melt together the coconut oil and chocolate. Remove from heat and

Stir in extracts of stevia. Add chopped peanuts. Using a spoon, drop over a parchment-lined pan and set aside until harden then put them in the fridge.

7.12 Coconut Macadamia Bars

Preparation time: 5 mins

Total time: 5 mins

 Calories327kcal

Ingredients

- almond butter half cup
- coconut oil one fourth cup
- macadamia nuts sixty grams
- Shredded coconut unsweetened six tablespoons
- Stevia drops twenty

Method

Crush by a food processor or by hand the macadamia nuts.

In a mixing bowl, add the coconut oil, almond butter, and shredded cocoa. Add the drops of stevia and macadamia nuts.

Mix thoroughly, and pour the batter into a baking dish lined with 99 parchment paper and chill overnight.

7.13 Almond Butter and Coconut balls

Preparation time: 5 mins

Total time: 5 mins

 Calories87kcal

Ingredients

- Vanilla almond whey protein one third cup

- almond butter two-third cup
- Chocolate chips sugar-free one cup
- Stevia drops a half teaspoon
- Flaked coconut unsweetened one cup

Method

Add all of the ingredients in a medium bowl until well combined.

Scoop about a tablespoon and shape into balls. Cover and place in the fridge.

7.14 Blackberry Coconut Fat Bombs –

Preparation time: 5 mins

Cooking time: 5 mins

Total time: 10 mins

Ingredients

- blackberries half cup
- Coconut butter one cup
- Stevia half teaspoon
- coconut oil one cup
- lemon juice one tablespoon
- Vanilla powder one fourth teaspoon

Method

Place coconut oil, coconut butter, and blackberries in a pan and heat over medium heat until well mixed. Add the coconut oil mixture and remaining ingredients to a food processor and blend until smooth.

Note: Separation may occur when a mixture of coconut oil is too dry. If fresh berries are used, cooking them with the coconut oil and butter is not required. Spread into a small pan lined with parchment paper and cool for one hour or until the mixture has hardened. Cut into squares and place the refrigerator, in a covered container

7.15 Maple Oatmeal

Prep Time5 minutes

Cook Time20 minutes

Total Time25 minutes

Protein: 9.25g

Net carbs: S3.27g

Fat: 34.59g

Ingredients

- Sunflower seeds one fourth cup
- Walnuts half cup
- Pecans half cup
- Coconut flakes one fourth cup
- Almond milk unsweetened four cups
- Chia seeds four tablespoons
- Cinnamon half teaspoon
- Stevia powder 3/8 teaspoon

- Maple flavor one teaspoon

Method

Put the pecans, walnuts, and sunflower seeds to a food processor and grind them. Put all the ingredients in a pan. Put on low heat and simmer until the chia seeds have absorbed much of the liquid, stirring for a good thirty minutes. Turn off the heat when the oatmeal has thickened, and serve warm. You can also let it cool down the next day and store it in the refrigerator for your breakfast.

7. 16 Tofu Feta

Preparation time: 5 minutes

Total time: 5 minutes

Servings: Eight

Calories: 69kcal

Ingredients

- basil one teaspoon

- oregano one teaspoon

- lemon juice one tablespoon

- firm tofu one tablespoon

- Olive oil extra virgin one tablespoon

- Nutritional yeast two tablespoons

- Pepper and salt to taste

Method

Mix all ingredients leaving out tofu.

Cut tofu into small pieces. Add the dressing over tofu and keep it overnight.

7.17 Chocolate Peanut Butter Smoothie

Preparation time: 5 minutes

Yield: 1 serving

Ingredients

- Cocoa powder unsweetened two teaspoons
- Coconut milk three fourth cup
- Avocado half
- Cinnamon powder one teaspoon
- Peanut butter one tablespoon
- Stevia to taste

Method

Mix all the above-mentioned ingredients in the blender and blend well.

Chapter 8: Freezable Keto Recipes

8.1 Keto breakfast cookies

Keto breakfast cookies soft, thick and chewy packed with wholesome low carb ingredients. We are vegan, eggless, paleo-free, gluten-free and sugar-free, ideal for preparing in advance and enjoying a quick breakfast

Course: Breakfast

Cuisine: American

Preparation time: 5 minutes

Cooking time: 18 minutes

Servings: 20 Cookies

Calories: 160kcal

Ingredients

- Half cup flour (coconut)
- Two tablespoon flaxseeds grounded
- 1 3/4 cup almond flour blanched
- One teaspoon cinnamon
- One and a half cup sweetener granulated (anyone)
- Three fourth cup softened coconut butter
- One cup of chocolate chips (keto)
- 1 1/4 cups butter (almond)
- Half cup coconut flakes shredded unsweetened
- Two tablespoon chia seeds grounded

Method

Mix ground chia seeds with five tablespoons of water in a small pot and place them aside until a gel is formed.

Combine the cinnamon, coconut flour, baking soda, almond flour, coconut flakes, unsweetened coconut flakes, and ground flaxseed in a large mixing bowl.

Put coconut oil, selected granulated sweetener, almond butter, and prepared chia eggs in a separate bowl, then blend until completely mixed.

Combine your both ingredients dry and wet, and mix well. Fold your chocolate chips through and cover your bowl and refrigerate for about an hour to cool the dough.

Then preheat your oven to 180C or 350F and line and set aside a large baking tray with parchment paper.

Shape 16-20 dough balls, and put them on the lined tray. Push each ball into a form of a cookie and bake for 15-18 minutes or until it is properly cooked from the center.

Take out the cookies tray from the oven and allow them to fully cool on the pan.

Tips on stocking and freezing

Storing in fridge

Keto breakfast cookies can keep well in a sealed container at room temperature for up to 3 days. Keeping the cookies refrigerated is best, as they will maintain their chewy texture and also keep for seven days.

Freezing

Breakfast cookies are freezer friendly and are great to freeze for the weeks/months ahead for easy grab-and-go breakfasts! Wrap cookies in parchment paper individually, and place them in a zip lock bag or shallow tub. Cookies will be kept frozen for at least six months.

To defrost them

Defrost them at room temperature the day before you intend to eat them. They can also be left overnight in the refrigerator.

8.2 Cinnamon Rolls

These simple and keto cinnamon rolls are a delicious low carb snack recipe! No cheese needed- Made with almond flour, they are fluffy, no cheese needed, and full of cinnamon flavor!

Preparation time: 10 minutes

Cooking time: 25 minutes

Servings: 14 Rolls

Calories: 174kca

Ingredients

- Three tablespoon tapioca flour
- Three cups almond flour
- One fourth teaspoon baking soda
- 1/2 tsp salt
- flex eggs
- Vanilla extract one teaspoon
- Granulated sweetener one fourth cup monk fruit, baking stevia, etc.
- One-fourth cup melted coconut oil
- Keto maple syrup two tablespoon
- Cinnamon two tablespoon

Method

Oven preheats to 180C/350F. Grease a baking dish lightly, or place parchment paper in it.

Combine the almond flour, tapioca flour, salt, and baking soda into a large dish. Whisk the coconut oil, the flax eggs, vanilla extract, and maple syrup together in a separate bowl.

Combine the ingredients dry and wet, and mix well. Form a ball, and set aside for 10 minutes.

Put a piece of parchment paper on a kitchen surface and sprinkle some almond flour over it, and put the dough ball on top. Sprinkle on top with more flour and place the second piece of parchment paper on top. Roll the dough into a square shape, around 1/4-1/2 inch thick, using a rolling pin.

Spread the coconut oil or butter over the top of the dough, until covered. Sprinkle with cinnamon and sugar, then add more as needed (the higher side you want). Carefully roll up the dough to hold it in place, using the parchment paper too. Refrigerate for a few minutes, when cleaning the oven.

Slice up the rolls of cinnamon and place them on the lined baking platter—Bake for 20-25 minutes, or to the top until golden.

Take out from the oven and frost.

Tips on Storage

To store: Keep the remaining cinnamon rolls in the refrigerator, in a sealable container. They're going to keep up to 5 days on well. Much longer, and the glaze becomes soggy.

To freeze: Cinnamon roll can only be frozen when it has not yet been frosted. Insert unfrosted rolls of cinnamon in a sealable container. They'll store well up to 6 months in the freezer.

Flax seeds replacement of eggs

The basic technique used to use flax as an egg replacement is clear and straightforward. Mix one tablespoon of finely ground flaxseed into three tablespoons of cold water for each egg that you are replacing. Set aside for five minutes so that the soluble fiber of the seeds can form its gel with the water.

8.3 Crispy Waffles

These soft and fluffy waffles are a balanced recipe for breakfasts, snacks, or even desserts, filled with protein. These simple low carb waffles are naturally gluten-free, paleo vegan, sugar-free, grain-free, and dairy-free, made with no butter, grains, oil, or sugar!

Ingredients

- One fourth cup oat flour
- Half scoop vanilla brown rice protein powder 17 grams
- Granulated sweetener one tablespoon
- flaxseeds grounded one tablespoon
- baking powder one fourth teaspoon
- Half cup non-dairy milk
- Vanilla extract one teaspoon

Method

Add your dry ingredients in a mixing bowl and set aside.

Add your flax, vanilla extract, baking powder, and one-fourth cup of milk in a separate bowl and whisk well and allow to sit for five minutes to start gelling.

Heat up the waffle iron, and combine the two bowls while it is heating up, add the extra one-fourth cup of milk until a thick batter is formed. Cook until all the batter is used on the waffle.

Once cooked, toast waffles in a toaster for crispier waffles.

Fluffy Crispy Keto waffles (Vegan, Paleo) are friendly to the freezer and can be frozen for later enjoyment. In parchment paper, wrap portions and place them in a zip lock bag.

Heat frozen waffles in a toaster.

8.4 Peanut Butter Cheesecake Bites

Yield: 16 cheesecake bites

Calories per serving: 140

Fat per serving: 6.2g

Carbs per serving: 2.g net

Protein per serving: 2.5g

Fiber per serving: 1.5g

Ingredients

- Vegan cream cheese eight tablespoons
- Vanilla extract one teaspoon
- Peanut butter eight tablespoons
- Stevia to taste

Method

Mix all the ingredients until they combined. Add about one-fourth teaspoon of liquid stevia, but you can add more if you like things on the sweeter side.

Place into liners. Freeze them for at least an hour.

8.5 Peanut Butter Pumpkin Pies

Yield: 4 mini pies

Serving Size: 1 mini pie

Calories per serving: 271

Fat per serving: 23g

Carbs per serving: 6.3g net

Protein per serving: 10.4g

Fiber per serving: 8.5g

Ingredients

For the Crust:

- One flax egg mix one tbsp. Flax seeds with 3 tbsp. water
- Coconut oil one fourth cup
- Coconut flour six tablespoons

For the Filling:

- Pumpkin puree a half cup
- Flax egg one
- peanut butter one fourth cup
- cinnamon one teaspoon
- granulated sweetener or lakanto one fourth cup

Method

Preheat an oven to 350F. Press the pie crust into four mini pie tins.

Mix the peanut butter, pumpkin, sweetener, cinnamon, and one flax egg together until well combined. Distribute the filling mixture evenly into the pie tray. Bake them for twenty minutes.

Use the leftover dough to cut small pumpkin shapes and bake those for 10 minutes, if you want to be fancy (when the little pies are baking). Top small pies with tiny pumpkins before the filling is fully set.

Take it out from the oven and let it cool before eating!

8.6 Chocolate Tofu Pudding

Preparation time: 5 mins

Total time: 5 mins

Ingredients

- cocoa powder unsweetened half cup

- tofu soft silken two pounds

- Monk fruit sweetener two tablespoons

- Vanilla extract half teaspoon

Method

Puree or blend all ingredients in a blender until smooth.

It can be prepared ahead and store in your frozen for three months.

8.7 Italian Baked Mushrooms

Preparation time: 10 minutes

Total time: 30 minutes

Protein14.3 grams

Net carbs5.9 grams

Fat16 grams

Calories231 kcal

Ingredients

- parmesan cheese one cup

- tomato one large

- Duck fat or ghee two tablespoons

- parsley, fresh one tablespoon

- salt and pepper to taste

- Mushrooms four
- Basil, fresh two tablespoons

- oregano dried one teaspoon

Method

Preheat your oven to 400 degrees Fahrenheit. Chop the mushrooms. Heat the ghee over medium flame in a non-stick pan. Add the chopped mushrooms, sprinkle salt and pepper, and cook for about five minutes. Take from heat and put the mushrooms in small baked dishes. Wash and chop the herbs. In a bowl, mix the parsley, basil, and tomatoes with the herbs and season with salt to taste. Top with grated parmesan cheese and put in a preheated oven for twenty-five minutes.

8.8 Apple Pie Protein Muffins

Preparation time: 5 minutes

Cooking time: 15 minutes

Total Time: 20 minutes

Servings: 15 muffins

Calories: 86kcal

Ingredients

- Baking powder one teaspoon
- Almond flour half cup
- Vanilla protein powder two scoops
- cinnamon, apple pie spice, nutmeg, and clove one teaspoon
- Almond butter half cup
- Apple sauce unsweetened half cup
- Coconut oil half cup

For the healthy glaze

- Granulated sweetener one tablespoon
- Coconut butter half cup
- Lemon juice one tablespoon
- Milk unsweetened one-fourth cup.

Method

Preheat the oven to 350 d Fahrenheit, and line and set aside a 16 count mini muffin box or regular muffin pan.

Add all your ingredients in a bowl or blender and mix until smooth.

The muffin batter is uniformly distributed in the lined muffin pan. Bake for 10-15 minutes, then test with a skewer at the 10-minute mark. If it comes out clean, then there are muffins. Allow 5 minutes to cool in the pan before transferring to a wire rack to completely cool. Pour glaze, pour over cooled muffins.

8.9 Thai Soup

Preparation time: 10 mins

Cooking time: 15 mins

Total time: 25 mins

Ingredients

- red bell pepper julienned half
- red onion julienned half
- mushrooms three sliced
- garlic two cloves chopped
- ginger root half-inch chopped
- tamari one tablespoon
- cilantro chopped a handful
- Thai chili half chopped
- Vegetable broth two cups
- Coconut milk 400ml
- Stevia sweetener one tablespoon
- Firm tofu, cubed ten oz.

- Lime juice half

Method

In a big pot put all vegetables (onion, red bell pepper, mushrooms, garlic, ginger, and Thai chili), broth, coconut milk, and sugar and boil. Cook for about five minutes over medium heat.

Add tofu and cook for an additional five minutes. Remove from heat, stir in tamari, lime juice, and fresh coriander. Hold the soup in the refrigerator in a sealed jar for up to 5 days. You can freeze that too.

8.10 Pizza Sticks

Preparation Time: 10 minutes

Cooking time: 30 mins

Total time: 40 mins

 Servings: Four servings

Ingredients

- tomato sauce one-fourth cup plus one tablespoon

- Firm tofu one block

- nutritional yeast two tablespoons plus two teaspoon

- dried basil a pinch

Tofu drain: roll tofu block into the paper towel and drain the tofu for 20 minutes.

Preheat oven to 425F as tofu is cooking, line baking sheet with parchment paper.

Cut tofu into 16 thin pieces and put on sheet baking. Spread 1 tsp of marinara sauce over each stick of the pizza. Sprinkle each stick with 1/2 tsp of nutritional yeast.

Sprinkle basil to taste, over tofu sticks.

Conclusion

In recent years, interest in the benefits of the ketogenic diet has pushed people, thus revealing health benefits like improved weight loss to safety against chronic conditions like diabetes and heart disease.

The ketogenic technique was originally established to reduce the effects of fasting by drastically reducing carb intake, which puts the body into ketosis. During ketosis, the body starts burning fat for energy, rather than relying on dietary carbohydrates for energy.

This process leads to a number of positive impacts on your health, with growing evidence suggesting that the keto diet can protect against certain neurological problems, aid in regulating insulin levels to lower symptoms of polycystic ovary syndrome, and even help prevent cancer cells from growing.

So how exactly do you fall into ketosis without taking butter and meat? Also, how can you make sure that your nutrient requirements are still being met while adopting a plant-based ketogenic diet?

The trick is to swap out your starchy vegetables for low-carb alternatives while also loading your diet with plenty of plant-based proteins and fats. This can help you stay under your carbohydrate goal and provide your body with the important minerals and vitamins that it needs to stay healthy.

www.ingramcontent.com/pod-product-compliance
Lightning Source LLC
Chambersburg PA
CBHW070808240726
48654CB00007B/259